Current Maxillofacial and Orthopedic Fracture Management - Techniques and Challenges

Edited by Mazen Ahmad Almasri and Sedeek M. Mosaid

Published in London, United Kingdom

Current Maxillofacial and Orthopedic Fracture Management - Techniques and Challenges
http://dx.doi.org/10.5772/intechopen.1009711
Edited by Mazen Ahmad Almasri and Sedeek M. Mosaid

Contributors
Alberto Jorge-Mora, Ashok Marudanayagam, Belen Ines Vieira-Lopez, Branislav Krivokapic, Diego Novillo-Casal, Einal Bathish, Fadi Abboud, Felipe Ignacio Vergara-Gutiérrez, Fernando Antunez-Muiños, Gergő Józsa, Haim Shtarker, Herman Nudelman, Iván Castro-Arias, Jelena Jadzic, Jorge González-García, Khalil Nasrallah, Milutin Micic, Murat Yüncü, Paul Lee, Rizwan Shahid, Sedeek M. Mosaid, Slavisa Zagorac, Tamara de la Rasilla-Sainz, Yousif Jihad

First published in London, United Kingdom, 2026 by IntechOpen
IntechOpen is the global imprint of INTECHOPEN LIMITED, registered in England and Wales, registration number: 11086078, 167-169 Great Portland Street, London, W1W 5PF, United Kingdom

For EU product safety concerns: IN TECH d.o.o., Prolaz Marije Krucifikse Kozulić 3, 51000 Rijeka, Croatia, info@intechopen.com or visit our website at intechopen.com.

British Library Cataloguing-in-Publication Data
A catalogue record for this book is available from the British Library

Current Maxillofacial and Orthopedic Fracture Management - Techniques and Challenges
Edited by Mazen Ahmad Almasri and Sedeek M. Mosaid
p. cm.
Print ISBN 978-1-83769-821-9
Online ISBN 978-1-83769-820-2
eBook (PDF) ISBN 978-1-83769-873-8

Meet the editors

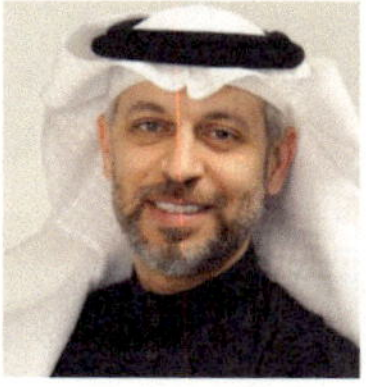

Professor Mazen A. Almasri is an Oral Maxillofacial Surgeon at King Abdulaziz University in Jeddah, Saudi Arabia. He is an active surgeon at the KAU Health Center and in private practice. Furthermore, an academic educator and a researcher. He pursued his clinical training in OMFS at McGill University (Montreal, Quebec, Canada), where he completed his master's degree and fellowship in implantology and reconstruction in 2010. Since 2009, he has been an active fellow of the Royal College of Canada and a diplomat of the American Board of OMFS (2011). Prof. Almasri's passion for managing maxillofacial deformities, dental implantology, and reconstruction has led him to publish numerous articles, chapters, and textbooks.

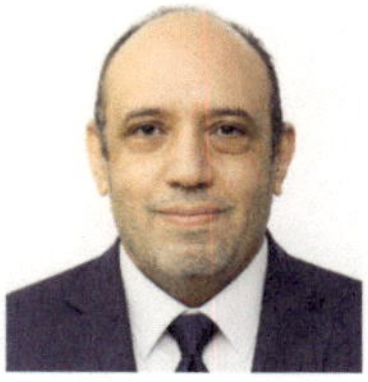

Dr. Sedeek M. Mosaid is a Senior Specialty Doctor in Trauma and Orthopedic Surgery at an NHS Trust in the UK. He holds FRCS (Trauma & Orthopedics) from the Royal College of Surgeons of Edinburgh and FRCS (Surgery) from the Royal College of Surgeons in Ireland. Dr. Mosaid is involved in medical education. He is a mentor in the RCSEd Surgical Mentoring Scheme. He has contributed to peer-reviewed publications and book chapters, and he is interested in orthopedic research and education. He remains engaged in supporting clinical practice and teaching within orthopedic surgery.

Contents

Preface

Orthopedic trauma surgery is undergoing rapid evolution, propelled by advances in biomechanics, biological understanding, and technological innovation. Contemporary fracture management now encompasses personalized approaches, advanced imaging modalities, and refined perioperative strategies to optimize patient outcomes. This edited volume, *Current Maxillofacial and Orthopedic Fracture Management - Techniques and Challenges*, compiles current perspectives on both foundational principles and complex clinical scenarios encountered in modern orthopedic practice.

The volume opens with an examination of the evolution of internal fixation in growing bones, emphasizing the shift from purely mechanical solutions to biologically informed strategies. It then discusses innovative orthopedic approaches utilizing computer-aided design and manufacturing, underscoring the expanding role of precision medicine in surgical planning and execution.

Subsequent chapters address fracture management in specific anatomical regions and patient populations. The challenges associated with acetabular fractures in elderly patients are analyzed, with particular attention to decision-making in this vulnerable group with complex comorbidities. The discussion then turns to spinal fractures, outlining current treatment options and emerging perspectives. This section concludes with a comprehensive overview of calcaneal fractures, detailing current diagnostic and management strategies.

The final section of the volume examines the most challenging aspects of orthopedic trauma care. Fracture nonunion persists as a significant clinical issue, necessitating a comprehensive understanding of both biological and mechanical factors. This discussion is complemented by a chapter on complicated fractures, which provides practical strategies for managing cases that require advanced surgical judgment and expertise.

Collectively, this volume is intended to offer clinicians, trainees, and researchers a concise yet comprehensive overview of contemporary concepts in fracture management. By integrating foundational knowledge with emerging innovations, the book aims to support evidence-based practice and foster continued progress in orthopedic trauma care.

We extend our sincere gratitude to all contributing authors for their expertise and dedication, as well as to the publishing team for their invaluable support throughout the development of this volume.

Mazen Ahmad Almasri
Oral Maxillofacial Surgery Department,
Faculty of Dentistry,
King Abdulaziz University,
Jeddah, Saudi Arabia

Sedeek M. Mosaid
Trauma and Orthopaedic Surgery,
NHS Trust,
United Kingdom

Section 1

Foundations and Innovations in Orthopaedics

Chapter 1

From Metal to Molecular: The Evolution of Internal Fixation in Growing Bones

*Herman Nudelman and Gergő Józsa**

Abstract

This chapter explores the paradigm shift in paediatric fracture management, tracing the evolution of internal fixation from traditional metallic hardware to modern biodegradable molecular implants. With a focus on growing bones, we discuss the limitations of rigid, permanent materials in paediatric populations and the emergence of bioabsorbable polymers – particularly PLGA (poly-lactic-co-glycolic acid) – as a safer, more adaptable alternative for certain cases. The chapter highlights clinical applications, MRI-based follow-up strategies, and absorption profiles. We also examine current trends in injury patterns among children, the impact of changing lifestyles and activities, and how emerging technologies such as 3D imaging and surgical planning are enhancing precision in treatment. Furthermore, other types of degradable implants (magnesium, zinc, PGA, PLA, etc.) will be mentioned as well. Practical considerations, including cost-effectiveness, complication rates, and regulatory implications, are addressed to provide a comprehensive overview of this rapidly advancing field.

Keywords: osteosynthesis, absorbable, fracture management, biodegradable implants, paediatric trauma

1. Introduction

The first recorded metal fixation occurred in 1775 with an iron wire described in a French manuscript. Widespread use had to wait for three developments: anesthesia (1846), antisepsis/asepsis (1867–1886), and X-rays (1896). Joseph Lister promoted safe open reduction and used metal wires himself.

Early innovators like Hansmann and Lane introduced metal plates and screws for bone stabilisation [1]. However, surgeons have exercised caution regarding internal fixation in children due to the distinctive challenges associated with the developing skeleton [2, 3]. Growth plates found within the developing skeleton make surgical fixation challenging [2]. Rigid implants could damage growth plates and disrupt normal growth. The risk of implant-related infections or soft-tissue irritation is also high, as hardware is left protruding [4, 5]. For most of the 20th century, paediatric fractures were treated conservatively with casting or traction. Internal fixation with screws or nails was typically reserved for more severe cases. As surgical techniques improved and complications became less worrisome, implants could be used on children too.

In the 1980s, an important improvement was introduced. Metaizeau and his colleagues in France developed elastic stable intramedullary nailing (ESIN). Inserting a titanium or steel rod with flexible slots into the medullary canal was thought to provide internal support and reduce surgical risks [6, 7]. The technique provided stable fixation through small incisions while avoiding crossing the growth plate [7]. Clinical adoption was fueled by its favourable outcomes, as treated children could often mobilise earlier and had lower complication rates than with traction or casting [8]. Even so, metallic implants carry their limitations: they are not absorbed and thus routinely require a second removal operation [5]. Additionally, metals can sometimes migrate or 'back out', occurring in roughly 5–12% of paediatric cases and leading to soft-tissue irritation or loss of fracture reduction [9, 10]. Infection risks are further increased due to implant migration, leading to discomfort [11, 12]. Hardware that protrudes through the skin may be predisposed to skin and soft tissue infections (SSTIs) [10, 11]. Even though metal implants offer reliable support, they require removal and can disrupt bone growth.

To address these concerns, orthopaedic research turned towards biodegradable fixation materials that could fulfil the mechanical requirements of an implant during healing but then safely dissolve [13]. Early investigations date back to the early 20th century. Notably, Lambotte reported the use of magnesium devices for fracture fixation, but it was not until the late 1980s that bioresorbable internal fixation became a clinical reality [14, 15]. In 1989, Böstman and colleagues in Finland published the first paediatric case series using bioabsorbable polymers to fix fractures across the growth plate [16]. Shortly thereafter, in 1991, a randomised trial by Hope *et al.* demonstrated that bioabsorbable pins could achieve outcomes equivalent to those of traditional K-wires in the fixation of children's elbow fractures [17]. Svensson *et al.* examined 50 cases of paediatric fractures treated with polyglycolic acid (PGA) rods and reported a 96% rate union [18]. When compared to metallic fixation, significant differences could not be found in alignment or function [18]. The primary benefit was apparent in reducing the need for routine hardware removal and its associated risks [13]. At the same time, further follow-up was needed, as a few polymer-specific complications were observed, including occasional foreign-body reactions that delayed healing [19]. These events highlighted that material biocompatibility and degradation behaviour would be critical considerations [20–22].

Over the following decades, polymer implants were formulated [23]. Biodegradable polymer implants may directly address the historical problems of migration, infection, and growth-plate disturbance [20, 24].

Initial polymer implants, however, had important limitations. PGA implants tended to lose strength relatively quickly and could induce a strong inflammatory response due to their acidic degradation byproducts [25]. PLA had a longer resorption time (often 2–3 years or more), maintaining strength longer, but the slow degradation sometimes led to late complications, such as sterile sinus tract formation or cystic changes, as the body reacted to retained polymer fragments [26–28]. In some cases, PLA degradation was so slow that implants persisted well beyond healing, causing irritation and requiring removal – defeating the purpose of using an absorbable device [25, 29]. Additionally, bioresorbable polymers are not osteoconductive; they do not actively promote bone healing, and, in fact, the localised acidic environment from degradation can cause temporary osteolysis (bone erosion) around the implant, depending on the degradation rate [20, 29]. Another issue was the mechanical strength of polymer implants. Early devices were not rigid enough to match the rigidity of metal, and the anticipated loss of strength could lead to fracture displacement before healing in load-bearing applications [30, 31]. As the bending (Young's) modulus of these implants is similar to that of bone, any force that would damage or fracture the bone will ultimately damage the implant [24, 32].

Copolymerisation of PGA and PLA yields PLGA, with tailored degradation mechanics [32]. By altering the composition, namely the L-lactide-to-glycolide ratio (generally 85 L:15 G), we can control the degradation rate [24]. Newer implants also include buffering and osteoconductive additives. For example, some PLGA implants include β-tricalcium phosphate (TCP) or hydroxyapatite particles [22, 26, 33]. These additives serve dual purposes: they make the polymer implants visible on X-ray (radio-opaque) and neutralise acidic byproducts, mitigating the local pH drop and stimulating bone ingrowth into the degrading implant's footprint [26, 33]. Thanks to these improvements, modern bioabsorbable implants cause far less inflammatory reaction and exhibit more controlled absorption, avoiding the extremes of excessively slow or rapid degradation seen with earlier devices [26]. The ultimate load-bearing capacity of PLGA remains lower than that of metals, limiting its use to low- and moderate-stress fractures [26].

Various types of implants are available for different purposes. Resorbable screws, available in standard and headless configurations, as well as cannulated or non-cannulated forms, can be inserted over a guidewire, ensuring accurate trajectory and minimising soft-tissue trauma. These are used for metaphyseal or epiphyseal fixation and osteochondral fragments, providing compression and low-profile stability suitable for intra-articular applications [34–39]. Intramedullary nails of varying lengths are typically used for diaphyseal fractures of the forearm or clavicle; the medullary canal is first prepared with smooth steel dilators, and the nail is gently progressed under fluoroscopic control. Forceful hammering must be avoided to prevent implant fracture. These nails are applied in long-bone fractures such as the forearm or clavicle, offering elastic, load-sharing support similar to traditional ESIN [22, 40]. Short IM nails are intended for smaller bones or metaphyseal regions, such as the distal radius, where buried fixation eliminates the risk of pin-site complications. These are usually inserted percutaneously, then cut at or just below the cortical surface to eliminate protrusion. Pins and rods may be used for tension-band constructs or small fragment fixation, while bioabsorbable plates, though less common, are available for specific anatomic reconstructions [17, 39, 41].

Recently, research focus has shifted towards biodegradable metals, specifically magnesium (Mg) alloys [23, 26]. Magnesium constructs could provide the strength of metal implants while being fully absorbable [14, 26]. New surface treatments and alloy designs can alter magnesium's rapid corrosion and enable its use as a safe temporary implant. As mentioned, magnesium's use in orthopaedics is a renaissance of an old idea; Albin Lambotte's early 1930s experiments using a Mg implant in bone were an antecedent of today's research [14, 15]. Current magnesium alloys (often containing rare-earth elements or zinc to improve stability) degrade at a controlled rate, releasing magnesium ions that the body's metabolic processes can assimilate. One early clinical milestone was a 2013 pilot study that used a fully bioabsorbable magnesium-alloy screw for hallux valgus surgery. Within 1 year, the screw had largely resorbed, and clinical outcomes were equivalent to those with a standard titanium screw fixation. Since then, orthopaedic applications of magnesium implants have broadened, including promising uses in paediatric patients. A systematic review and series by Baldini et al. on the use of resorbable magnesium screws in children for various fracture and osteotomy cases found complete bone healing without any implant-related complications, no growth disturbances, or device failure on short-term follow-up [34, 42]. Notably, there was no need to remove hardware, as Mg screws gradually dissolved [42]. Early results suggest that magnesium-based fixation could effectively address many traditional concerns [34]. Moreover, degradable metals may offer higher initial strength than polymers, potentially extending the use of absorbable implants to larger load-bearing applications in adolescents that were previously only amenable to permanent metal fixation [26, 34].

2. Advances from metallic to resorbable implants

2.1 Forearm fractures

Both-bone forearm fractures (radius and ulna) are among the most common paediatric long-bone injuries [30]. Operative fixation is indicated when there is displacement with angulation >15°, rotation >45° in children below the age of 10, and angulation >10°, rotation >30° in children above 10, complete displacement, open fractures, compartment syndrome, bayonet apposition above the age of 10 and from 1 cm, or instability after closed reduction, particularly in older children approaching skeletal maturity [43, 44]. ESIN has long been the gold standard for such cases, providing stable internal splinting through a minimally invasive approach that preserves the periosteum and growth plate integrity. ESIN achieves high union rates and allows early mobilisation; however, metal nail ends may irritate soft tissue or migrate (reported in 5–12% of cases), occasionally compromising reduction or causing discomfort. PLGA implants are inserted analogously to ESIN – via minor metaphyseal entry points under fluoroscopic guidance – and provide sufficient elastic stability for diaphyseal fractures in the skeletally immature [40]. RINs retain mechanical integrity for the first months, coinciding with the critical phase of callus formation, and subsequently undergo gradual hydrolytic degradation over 1–2 years [30, 44]. The resorption profile mirrors healing, allowing the implant to maintain support during consolidation and then to disappear without removal, as it is replaced by bone tissue [22, 30, 44].

Recent case series and retrospective and prospective studies report uneventful bone union and complete restoration of pronation–supination within 1 year of PLGA fixation, outcomes comparable to those with titanium ESIN [40, 45]. Secondary surgery due to implant failure was a result of repeated falls. Typically, adverse events are rare and self-limited but may include a mild inflammatory reaction, swelling, or transient entry-site irritation during polymer breakdown [22, 30, 40, 45]. Due to their radiolucency, β-tricalcium phosphate (TCP) tips have been incorporated as markers to enhance intraoperative and postoperative visualisation, a necessary adaptation to ensure accurate positioning (**Figure 1**). Surgeons should perform thorough canal preparation and careful insertion, as PLGA implants are more sensitive to torsion, hammering, and bending than metal. Technical challenges may

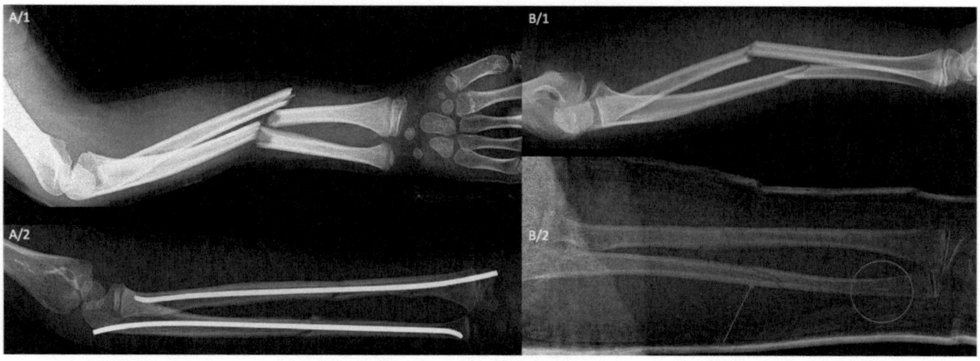

Figure 1.
Comparative forearm fracture fixation in a child. A: both-bone forearm fracture (a/1-preop X-ray), stabilised with traditional ESIN (metal rods visible within the medullary canals – A/2). B: a similar fracture (B1 – preop image) treated with two PLGA intramedullary nails (radiopaque TCP markers are highlighted by the pink circle; on the otherwise radiolucent polymer nails are indicated by the arrow).

arise in small children, whose medullary canals are relatively narrow. A temporary external splint or short cast is recommended to supplement fixation until callus formation begins. Long-term follow-up demonstrates that by 18–24 months, PLGA nails are radiographically absent and replaced by remodelled bone without residual voids or osteolysis [22, 40, 46]. Overall, bioabsorbable intramedullary nails reproduce the mechanical principles of ESIN – three-point fixation and elastic stability – while eliminating the burden of hardware removal and the associated complications of metallic nails. Studies have yielded comparable results regarding efficacy, safety, and healing [30, 40, 47].

2.2 Clavicle fractures

Mid-shaft clavicle fractures account for the majority of paediatric clavicular injuries. While most heal uneventfully with conservative management, operative fixation is absolutely indicated when there is an open fracture, subclavian vein or artery injury, floating shoulder, complete displacement, > 2 cm of shortening, skin tenting, or symptomatic malalignment, particularly in active adolescents [48]. The traditional surgical approach employs ESIN, using a flexible titanium or stainless-steel nail introduced retrograde through the sternal end of the clavicle; however, plates can also be utilised [49, 50]. This method preserves periosteal continuity, minimises soft-tissue stripping, and yields high union rates. Nevertheless, metallic nails frequently cause hardware prominence and skin irritation over the thin subcutaneous clavicle, sometimes accompanied by migration of the nail tip [48, 50]. Because of these issues and the need to prevent interference with clavicular growth, implant removal is routinely required several months after union, adding anaesthesia exposure and potential refracture risk at the entry site [48, 50].

The technique with RIN is identical. Via a small medial entry point, the nail is inserted along the medullary canal under fluoroscopic guidance [50]. Incorporated TCP tips aid intraoperative visualisation and positioning. During insertion, gentle rotation rather than hammering is advised. Avoid over-bending the implant and ensure the correct diameter. A period of brief immobilisation using a sling is recommended (**Figure 2**). Early institutional experience and a few clinical cases have

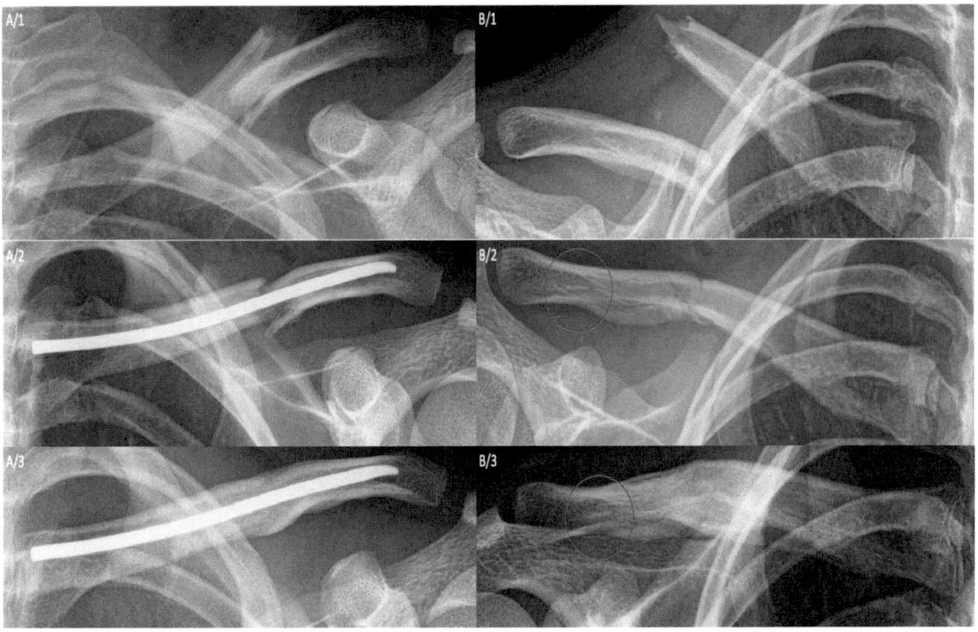

Figure 2.
Intramedullary fixation of a midshaft clavicle fracture. Panel A shows a paediatric clavicle fracture stabilised with a traditional titanium ESIN. Panel B shows a similar fracture fixed with a ***bioabsorbable PLGA nail****. A1/B1 displays the pre-op imaging, while A2/B2 shows the results of fixation one day post-op. Follow-up images after – – corresponding to A3/B3 show healing and callus formation. The TCP tip is highlighted by the pink oval for better visualisation.*

demonstrated solid union, correct length restoration, and full shoulder function following PLGA nail fixation of displaced mid-shaft fractures. Radiographic follow-up described continuous callus formation and signs of remodelling within 3–6 months. Implant migration or soft-tissue irritation has not been noted institutionally. These outcomes are comparable to metals, yet with reduced postoperative discomfort [50].

2.3 Distal radius fractures

Fractures of the distal radius are the most common paediatric fractures, accounting for nearly one-third of all upper-extremity injuries [51–53]. Often, closed reduction and casting are sufficient. However, operative fixation is indicated when displacement exceeds 15–20 degrees of angulation, displacement over 2 mm, radial shortening over 5 mm, associated ulnar fracture, translation > 50%, or recurrent loss of reduction after manipulation – particularly in older children approaching skeletal maturity [54]. Kirschner wire (K-wire) pinning uses smooth stainless-steel wires, which are drilled percutaneously across the fracture [51]. Wire ends are left protruding through the skin for later removal. While this method is reliable, it carries several drawbacks. Exposed wire ends frequently irritate soft tissue, require daily pin-site care, and predispose patients to pin-tract infection (up to 8%) [55, 56]. Secondary removal of the wires, typically at 4–6 weeks post-injury, is obligatory and often uncomfortable. Absorbable short IM nails are introduced percutaneously through a small entry at the distal metaphysis and inserted into the medullary canal

[57]. Once the desired reduction is achieved, the implant is cut at or slightly below the cortical surface, leaving no external component (**Figure 3/A** and **B**). The nail diameter should ensure gentle canal filling. Supplemental immobilisation in a short-arm cast is recommended until early callus formation. Union rates exceeding 95%, without cases of implant migration, infection, or secondary displacement when short IM nails were used [57]. Overall complication rates were lower, and functional recovery and range of motion mirrored those seen after metallic K-wire fixation. Radiographs at 6 weeks typically show callus formation bridging the fracture without residual lucency, cystic change, or growth disturbance after one and a half years [57]. Based on limited available information, short bioabsorbable intramedullary nails can achieve stabilisation comparable to that of K-wires in paediatric distal radius fractures [57]. They effectively remove two key drawbacks of metal fixation, pin-tract infection and the mandatory removal procedure, while preserving minimally invasive principles [57].

2.4 Distal humerus: Lateral condylar and medial epicondylar fractures

Fractures around the distal humerus account for nearly one-tenth of paediatric elbow injuries and demand precise anatomic reduction to prevent long-term deformity or stiffness [58]. Lateral condyle fractures, typically Salter–Harris IV lesions extending into the articular surface, require operative fixation when displacement exceeds 2 mm, articular incongruity is questionable, or closed reduction fails to maintain alignment [59, 60]. Operative indications for medial

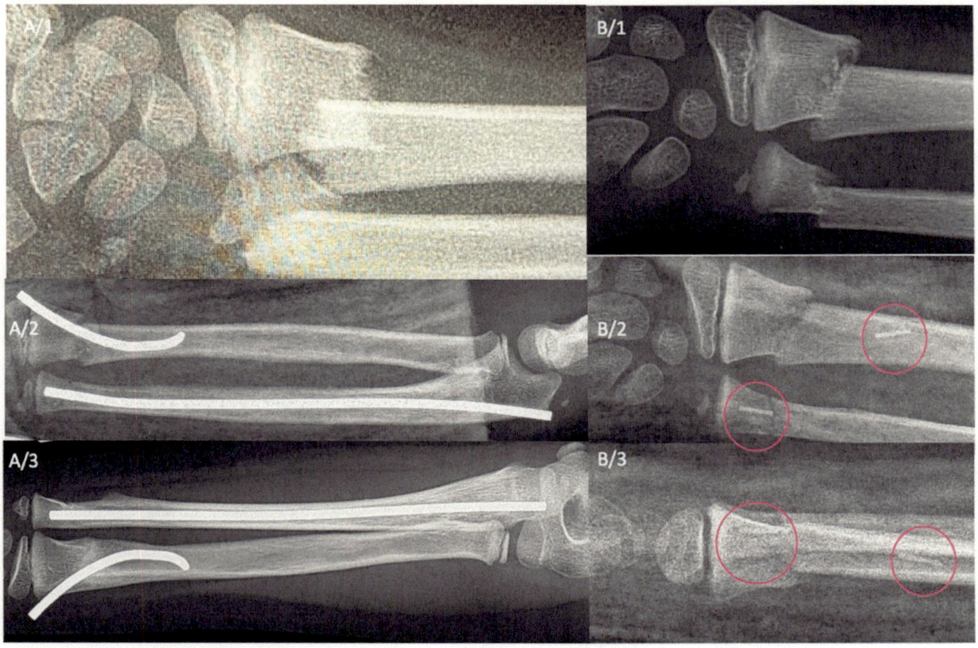

Figure 3.
Fixation of a paediatric distal radius fracture. Preop X-ray of the fracture (A/1). Results of conventional treatment with ulnar ESIN and a short titanium nail can be seen in A/2 and 3. Fixation with bioabsorbable short intramedullary nails. B/1 displays the pre-op AP view of the fracture, while B/2 and 3 show the correction by RIN. TCP tips are highlighted in the pink circles.

epicondylar fractures include displacement of more than 5–15 mm, associated elbow dislocation, ulnar-nerve compression, entrapment, valgus instability, or an open fracture [61]. Generally, partially threaded cannulated metal screws or multiple K-wires can be used [60]. The hardware often protrudes into the soft tissue, causing irritation, and removal is mandatory once healing is complete to avoid growth-plate tethering or implant migration [62, 63]. K-wires protruding through the skin also carry an infection risk and may hinder early joint motion – an important factor in elbow rehabilitation [62]. Absorbable screws and pins provide an elegant alternative. First, stabilisation with K-wires takes place. After articular congruity has been achieved, wires are replaced with absorbable screws/pins (**Figure 4**) Clinical reports demonstrate good results with bioabsorbable fixation in the paediatric elbow [64]. In small osteochondral fragments, the headless variant offers improved surface congruity. Because the implants gradually lose stiffness, early protected motion is permitted, but excessive stress loading should be avoided for six weeks. The overall learning curve is modest for surgeons accustomed to screw fixation. In both lateral condyle and medial epicondyle fractures, PLGA fixation can achieve radiographic and functional outcomes equivalent to those of metal screws or K-wires, while sparing the patient a secondary removal procedure [64, 65].

2.5 Olecranon fractures

Olecranon fractures, though relatively uncommon in children, occur as isolated avulsion injuries or as components of complex elbow fracture–dislocations [66]. Operative fixation is indicated when there is >2 mm displacement, loss of extensor continuity, or intra-articular incongruity that cannot be reduced [66–68]. Among options for operative management is tension-band wiring (TBW) [66, 67]. This includes the drilling of two parallel K-wires from the apex of the olecranon to the ulnar shaft and using steel wires looped to provide compression at the fracture line [68]. However, in children, the prominence of metallic hardware beneath thin subcutaneous tissue frequently causes irritation or pain, and pin migration or skin breakdown can occur [39, 68]. Two bioabsorbable pins are inserted across the olecranon fracture in the same trajectory as traditional wires, followed by passage of the PDS cord through a transverse ulnar drill hole and around the pin heads in a figure-of-eight pattern. This configuration recreates the compression dynamics of conventional TBW while being entirely absorbable. PLGA pins will maintain structural support, and the PDS loop retains tension during callus formation. Knot

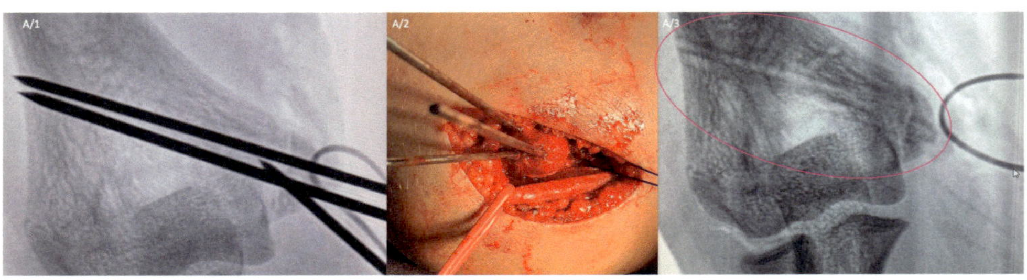

Figure 4.
Internal fixation of paediatric elbow fractures – medial epicondylar fracture. A/1 displays the intra-op fluoroscopic image of temporary k-wire stabilisation. A/2 displays an intra-op image of the fragment stabilised with k-wires. A3 highlights the resorbable pin encircled by the pink oval.

security with PDS is essential, as loss of tension may jeopardise compression. A recent clinical series of three patients demonstrated complete radiographic union, full restoration of range of motion, and absence of complications at one-year follow-up [39]. No inflammatory reactions or implant failures were observed, and – most importantly, no secondary surgery was required (**Figure 5**). Functional outcomes matched those of metallic constructs, while patient comfort and cosmetic satisfaction were improved [39].

2.6 Osteochondral fracture fixation in the knee: Lateral condyle and patella

Lateral condyle osteochondral lateral femoral condylar fractures are rare, often resulting from sports-related trauma or lateral patellar dislocation [69, 70]. Operative fixation is indicated when the fragment is displaced more than 2–3 mm, is large enough, or is symptomatic due to instability within the joint [71]. Nowadays, headless metallic compression screws or K-wires are used, depending on fragment size and location. Complications include cartilage abrasion and prominence-related irritation [72]. Recent clinical experience supports the reliability of the method with polymer implants. In a report, complete radiographic union and a standard range of motion within one year, with no need for hardware removal, was achieved [65]. Reduction was achieved and temporarily held with K-wires before definitive fixation with multiple resorbable nails [65]. Restoration of articular congruity is of the highest importance. After provisional stabilisation with K-wires, absorbable pins/

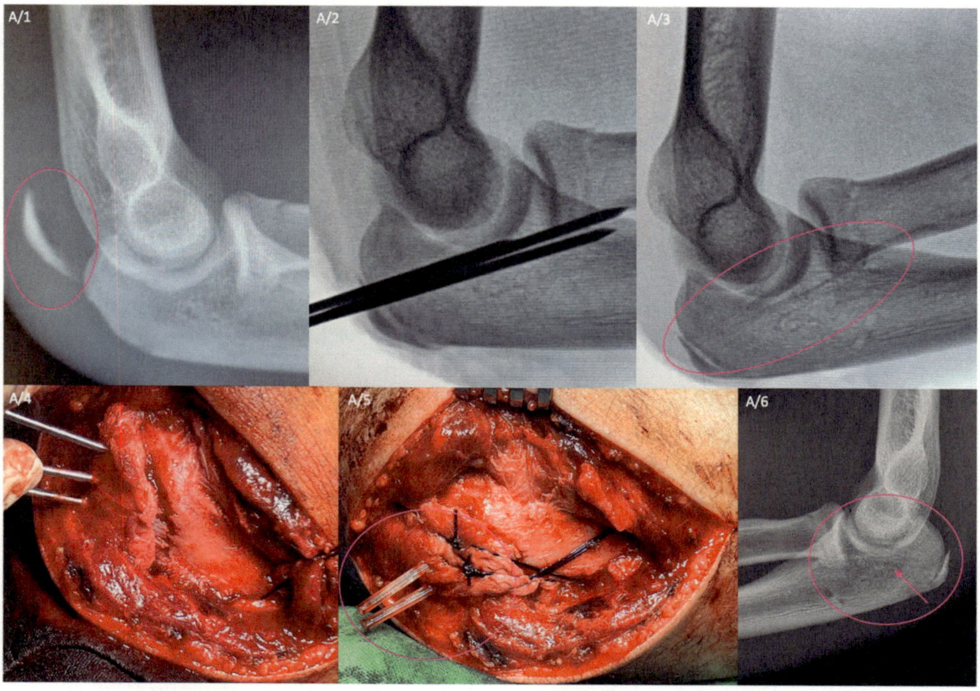

Figure 5.
A/1 displays the fragmented olecranon. A/2 shows the stabilisation with k-wires. A/3 displays the applied resorbable pins. A/4 shows intra-op images of the applied k-wire stabilisation. A/5 shows tension-band wiring with PDS loops and PLGA pins protruding before final clipping. A/6 displays post-op images, with the implant canal highlighted by the pink circle and arrow.

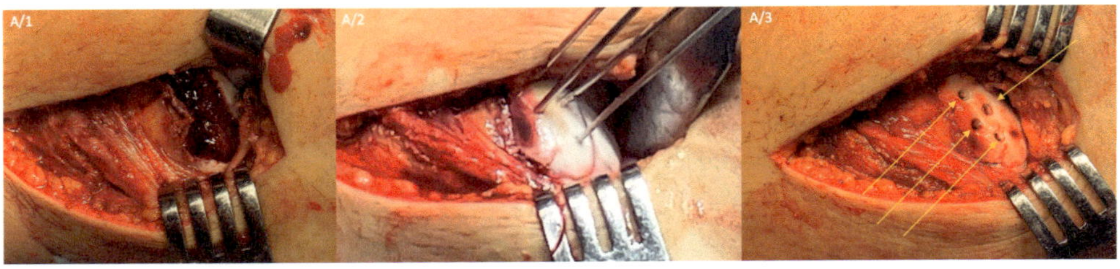

Figure 6.
Intra-op images of the defect (A/1), temporary K-wire stabilisation (A/2), and final fixation with resorbable pins (A/3).

nails should be inserted, ensuring compression without violating adjacent cartilage (**Figure 6**). Implants are countersunk 1–2 mm below the cortical surface to protect the surroundings. Early passive motion is recommended to prevent stiffness. Until radiographic evidence of union, weight-bearing is not permitted, typically around six weeks [35, 41, 71]. The gradual substitution of the resorbing implant by native bone has been verified by CT [65, 73].

2.6.1 Patella

Patellar osteochondral fractures are uncommon but clinically significant, as they often develop due to acute lateral patellar dislocation or direct trauma to the anterior knee [74, 75]. An osteochondral fragment is composed of cartilage and subchondral bone. Timely anatomic reduction is crucial in order to restore joint congruity and prevent long-term chondromalacia [74, 75]. Indications for surgical fixation include displacement over 2–3 mm, open fractures, articular step-off over 2–3 mm, loose bodies, or if the fragment is large enough to damage the articular surface [76]. Traditionally, fixation is achieved using metallic K-wires, small headless screws, or tension-band wiring for larger fragments [75–77]. Protrusion into the joint cavity, abrasion of the opposing cartilage, migration, and irritation of surrounding soft tissues are the main drawbacks [75]. Clinical series using resorbable pins for fixation have reported varying outcomes with minimal complications (**Figure** 7) [41]. Follow-up MRI imaging confirms fragment integration and gradual implant resorption after 12–18 months. However, when using PLA, pins were visible at the three-year follow-up [41]. Clinically, bioabsorbable fixation may offer union rates and functional recovery equivalent to metallic fixation. The ability to restore a smooth cartilage surface without long-term foreign material reduces the risk of postoperative irritation and mechanical abrasion [35, 41, 71] (**Table 1**).

3. Comparative outcomes and future perspectives

Clinical outcomes across anatomical sites provide evidence of success when using biodegradables [36, 38, 42, 78, 79]. High union rates and excellent functional recovery can be achieved in forearm and clavicle fractures by utilising RIN (resorbable IM nailing) [22, 40, 45, 47, 57]. Ankle fractures are among the most thoroughly studied applications. Paediatric patients treated with biodegradables experienced fewer complications and significantly shorter hospital stays, as reported in a 2024 study [36, 80, 81]. Clinical outcomes equivalent to those of metal fixation

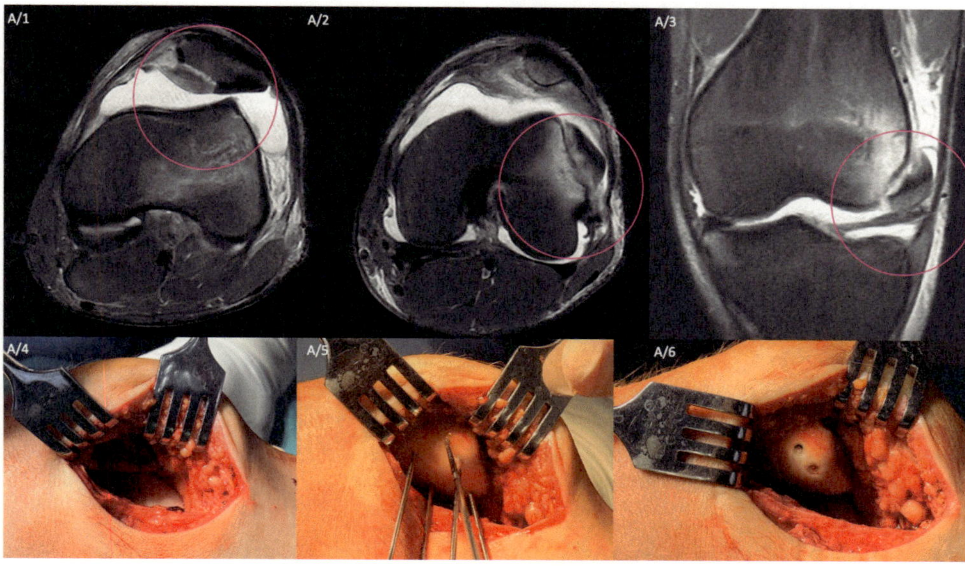

Figure 7.
The lesion and the fragment can be seen on MRI, highlighted by the pink circle (A/1, 2, and 3). Intraop images of the defect (A/4), temporary stabilisation with k-wires (A/5), and final fixation with absorbable implants (A/6).

were reported in adult ankle fractures [78, 81]. Forearm fractures in paediatric populations show excellent evidence, with randomised controlled trials confirming that bioabsorbable IM nails achieve equivalent outcomes to metal IM nails with notably fewer complications. Distal radius fractures were treated with short IM nails and achieved union rates exceeding 95% with minimal implant migration [57]. Medial epicondylar and lateral condylar fractures have also had promising results [42, 64]. Adult scaphoid fractures treated with bioabsorbable magnesium compression screws demonstrated high union rates with minimal complications [82–84]. A meta-analysis of 27 randomised controlled trials didn't find a statistically significant overall difference between the complication rates of absorbable (15.5%) and metallic implants (13.3%). However, newer materials demonstrated lower rates, with magnesium implants at 5%, without foreign body reactions in recent trials [85]. When examined by specific complication domain, absorbable implants demonstrated distinct advantages: experimental studies showed lower infection susceptibility, reductions in reoperation for removal, and virtual elimination of stress shielding complications due to biomechanical properties comparable to bone [42, 85–87]. In intra-articular fractures of the knee and osteochondral fragments, outcomes with absorbable pins are at least on par with metal [39, 41, 65, 71, 88].

PLGA in the 85 L:15 G composition demonstrated advantages over both metals and alternative absorbable polymers. Implants maintain full mechanical integrity for around eight weeks before undergoing complete degradation within approximately two years [36, 78–81]. Compared to previous absorbable polymers, PLGA represents an important milestone. The problem with polyglycolic acid (PGA) is that it degrades rapidly within 4 months, with mechanical strength loss after 6 weeks, and produces acidic byproducts that trigger intense inflammatory reactions. PLA implants, which degrade over 2-3 + years, are known for late complications, namely osteolysis (bone resorption around the implant) and cystic cavitation. Radiographic

Location	Implant type	Key technical pearls	Cautions/Common pitfalls
Forearm (Both-Bone)	Intramedullary nails (PLGA)	Prepare the canal with smooth dilators; insert nails by gentle rotation for three-point fixation; confirm radial head reduction before closure.	Avoid hammering; incorrect diameter selection may cause nail fracture or inadequate fixation.
Clavicle	Intramedullary nail (PLGA)	Insert retrograde through the sternal end under fluoroscopy; countersink the entry point slightly; maintain short sling immobilisation.	Over-insertion may cause medial perforation; excessive bending can fracture the nail. Reposition might require an open approach.
Distal Radius	Short intramedullary nails or pins (PLGA)	Insert percutaneously and cut flush with cortex; rely on TCP tip markers for fluoroscopic guidance; apply a cast for 1 week and utilise an orthosis for 3 more.	Do not leave the implant protruding; poor depth control increases soft-tissue irritation risk.
Distal Humerus – Lateral Condyle	PLGA screw or pin	Achieve anatomic reduction; insert screw perpendicular to fracture line; use headless type in intra-articular cases.	Excess torque can damage the polymer or fragment; avoid intra-articular protrusion.
Distal Humerus – Medial Epicondyle	PLGA screw or pin (depending on fragment size)	Reduce fragment anatomically; ensure gentle insertion; consider a headless design for smaller fragments.	Over-tightening risks physis violation; insufficient compression may cause nonunion. Watch for ulnar nerve
Olecranon	Two PLGA pins + PDS suture (resorbable tension-band)	Recreate figure-of-eight tension band; tie secure knots for sustained compression; start gentle motion after 2 weeks.	Loose knots can reduce fixation strength; ensure no suture entrapment under skin.
Patella	PLGApins or nails (1.5–2 mm)	Insert perpendicularly to the fragment and countersink below the cartilage; verify stability arthroscopically; begin early passive ROM.	Shallow placement risks cartilage abrasion; deep insertion may compromise compression.
Lateral Femoral Condyle	PLGA pins or nails (1.5–2 mm)	Reduce fragment anatomically; place multiple divergent pins for stability; countersink 1–2 mm beneath the surface.	Avoid excessive torque; delay weight-bearing until radiographic union (~6 weeks).

Table 1.
Summarises the practical considerations for applying bioabsorbable implants in common paediatric fracture sites. For each anatomical region, the preferred implant type, recommended intraoperative technique, and common pitfalls are listed.

examination in some series has shown osteolysis in over 50% of patients with tissue reactions [20, 26, 27, 85, 89]. In contrast, PLGA demonstrates excellent biocompatibility with minimal inflammatory response. PLGA IM nails demonstrated lower overall complication rates when compared to metal [22, 30, 40, 45]. The elastic modulus of 2-4 GPa versus titanium's ~ 110 GPa more closely approximates those of cortical bone, potentially reducing stress-shielding and implant loosening [23, 26, 89]. Recent evidence demonstrates that PLGA implants eliminate the need for secondary removal surgery, reduce radiation exposure and general anaesthesia burden in paediatric patients, and may provide clinical advantages through controlled micro-motion that enhances secondary bone healing and callus formation. The current literature indicates that PLGA is increasingly recognised as a viable alternative to metal implants for specific applications, particularly in paediatric populations [26, 30, 85].

Physicians need to be aware of the trade-offs of polymer materials, such as lower ultimate strength, risk of insertion failure, progressive loss of strength during degradation, the restriction to low-load applications, and possible material costs [23, 24, 32]. This necessitates accurate surgical technique and case selection. An anatomic reduction is essential (since there is limited opportunity for hardware-assisted late correction), and sufficient implants should be used to share the load during the healing process. Surgery should be supplemented with temporary casting or bracing to protect the repair during the early phase [26, 30, 40]. There remain scenarios where metallic fixation is still preferred: a length-unstable femoral shaft fracture, patients with high BMI, or a very proximal fracture with a short segment [23, 26]. In such cases, the superior strength of steel or titanium and the ability to bear full weight immediately can justify using a traditional implant. As many polymer implants are radiolucent, standard X-rays may not show the implant clearly. Radiopaque markers, such as β-tricalcium phosphate stripes in PLGA IM nails, are helpful to visualise implant position but these are not available for all implant types [40]. Degradation has been evaluated by Hedelin et al., describing over 90% absorption over a year with implant canals filled with bone [46]. Overall, the complications specific to bioabsorbables have been infrequent and generally mild. Transient inflammatory reactions or sterile fluid collections can occur in a small subset of cases as the polymer degrades, but these usually resolve without intervention. Long-term follow-up thus far (beyond 1–2 years) has not shown any late adverse sequelae like growth disturbances or osteolysis, but continued surveillance is prudent as larger cohorts of patients are observed into skeletal maturity [22, 40, 57, 90].

Biodegradable metal implants, such as those made from magnesium (Mg), are destined to further expand the capabilities of resorbable fixation. Magnesium has emerged as a notable alternative because it behaves more like a metal in terms of mechanical strength, yet it can corrode safely in the body [26, 91]. Implants are often alloyed with trace elements like zinc and yttrium to optimise the corrosion rate. During degradation, they release magnesium ions, which can stimulate bone formation and integration [26]. However, the degradation process for Mg produces a byproduct of hydrogen gas, which can form small radiolucent bubbles on X-ray around the implant [26, 91]. These postoperative gas pockets may form as a typical sign of magnesium resorption rather than being misinterpreted as an infection or osteolysis [26]. Over a period of months, if the amount of gas is negligible, it may dissipate, and the implant is progressively replaced by new bone [26, 91]. If the degradation rate is too fast and dubious amounts of gas are formed, as was the case with early, pure Mg implants, that could lead to severe consequences. Follow-up studies in children with Mg screws show that these radiographic lucent zones typically resolve by 6–12 months as bone healing progresses [91]. The sites where the screws were tend to ossify as the metal is absorbed [91]. Magnesium constructs offer higher initial strength than polymers. Laboratory pull-out tests have found that Mg screws have superior holding strength compared to PLA/PLGA screws and even rival stainless steel in some scenarios [26]. Another unique advantage is that magnesium is osteoconductive: as the surface of an Mg implant degrades, it can foster new bone growth directly onto it [26]. Though Young's modulus is closer to bone than that of titanium, evaluation of stress shielding and outcomes of load-sharing still needs to be investigated [26, 91].

Early clinical experience with magnesium implants in children has been highly encouraging. A 2022 systematic review summarised results from paediatric cases involving Mg screws used for various indications (fractures, osteotomies, and osteochondral defect fixations) [34]. The review reported excellent healing in nearly all cases, with union rates comparable to traditional metal fixation and no cases of implant-related growth arrest or systemic toxicity [34]. Specific comparative studies have also been published. In displaced medial epicondyle fractures of the humerus, a headless magnesium compression screw was compared with the standard two-K-wire technique [42]. The magnesium group (n = 12) had zero infections versus two deep infections in the K-wire group (n = 15) and one nonunion versus three fibrous nonunions with K-wires. Functionally, both groups did well, but the Mg screw patients avoided any hardware protrusion during healing and did not require removal under anaesthesia. By early 2025, regulatory approvals expanded worldwide raising confidence in safety and efficacy. A new magnesium screw system gained FDA authorisation in 2023 and CE Mark in 2025, with indications spanning from elbow to certain ankle fractures and applications in foot osteotomies [92].

The trend in orthopaedics is moving away from permanent metallic hardware towards implants that resorb. The evolution from metal to polymeric and now bio-metallic fixation is driven by the need to reduce implant-related morbidity. By providing reliable stability for the time that bone needs to heal and then gradually integrating or vanishing, these modern implants minimise interference with the patient's growth and tissues. The clinical evidence across forearm, clavicle, elbow, and knee injuries already shows that outcomes are equal, and sometimes superior, with bioresorbable implants. As technology evolves, we anticipate broader use and new indications for resorbable implants, ultimately making fracture treatments less invasive, not only at the time of surgery but over the entire course of healing. The advent of bioresorbable implants, from PGA and PLA to PLGA and magnesium, is bringing us ever closer to that ideal in fracture fixation.

4. Conclusion

In summary, the armamentarium for fracture fixation has dramatically expanded. Biodegradables may now achieve results equal to metal implants. As research continues, biodegradable implants will further broaden in indications, potentially handling more complex fractures and even being used for guided growth modulation or other innovative applications. The ultimate goal is improved healing with minimal morbidity, and these new materials and techniques are bringing that goal within reach, one resorbable implant at a time.

Conflict of Interest

The authors declare no conflict of interest.

Author details

Herman Nudelman[1,2*] and Gergő Józsa[1,2]

1 Division of Surgery, Traumatology, and Otorhinolaryngology, Department of Paediatrics, Clinical Complex, University of Pécs, Pécs, Hungary

2 Department of Thermophysiology, Institute for Translational Medicine, Medical School, University of Pécs, Pécs, Hungary

*Address all correspondence to: nuhwaao.pte@tr.pte.hu

References

[1] Hernigou P, Pariat J. History of internal fixation (part 1): Early developments with wires and plates before World War II. International Orthopaedics. 2017;**41**:1273–1283. DOI: 10.1007/s00264-016-3347-4

[2] Pretell-Mazzini J, Zafra-Jimenez JA, Rodriguez Martin J. Clinical application of locked plating system in children: An orthopaedic view. International Orthopaedics. 2010;**34**:931–938. DOI: 10.1007/s00264-010-0960-5

[3] Cundy PJ, Williams N. Metal implants in children. Journal of Children's Orthopaedics. 2024;**18**:557–568. DOI: 10.1177/18632521241293954

[4] Allen H, Davis KW, Noonan K, Endo Y, Nguyen JC. Orthopaedic fixation devices used in children: A radiologist's guide. Seminars in Musculoskeletal Radiology. 2018;**22**: 12–24. DOI: 10.1055/s-0037-1609013

[5] Montgomery BK, Gamble JG, Kha ST, Hecht GG, Vorhies JS, Lucas JF. Indications for and risks associated with implant removal after pediatric trauma. JAAOS Global Research and Reviews. 2022;6e2200050. DOI: 10.5435/JAAOS Global-D-22-00050

[6] Metaizeau JP, Ligier JN. Surgical treatment of fractures of the long bones in children. Interference between osteosynthesis and the physiological processes of consolidation. Therapeutic indications. Journal de Chirurgie. 1984;**121**:527–537

[7] Ligier JN, Metaizeau JP, Prévot J, Lascombes P. Elastic stable intramedullary nailing of femoral shaft fractures in children. The Journal of Bone and Joint Surgery. British Volume. 1988;**70**:74–77. DOI: 10.1302/0301-620X.70B1.3339064

[8] Duan L, Canavese F, Li L. Flexible intramedullary nails or Spica casting? A meta-analysis on the treatment of femur fractures in preschool children aged 2–5 years. Journal of Pediatric Orthopaedics B. 2023;**32**:292–301. DOI: 10.1097/BPB.0000000000001003

[9] Widjaja AB, Eng K, Griffiths J. Complications of internal fixation in paediatric fractures. ANZ Journal of Surgery. 2007;**77**:873–876. DOI: 10.1111/j.1445-2197.2007.04262.x

[10] Nisar A, Bhosale A, Madan SS, Flowers MJ, Fernandes JA, Jones S. Complications of Elastic Stable Intramedullary Nailing for treating paediatric long bone fractures. Journal of Orthopaedics. 2013;**10**:17–24. DOI: 10.1016/j.jor.2013.01.003

[11] Momaya A, Baker D, Gilbert S, Ponce B. Risk factors for complications and readmission after operative fixation of pediatric femur fractures. Journal of Children's Orthopaedics. 2015;**9**:307–311. DOI: 10.1007/s11832-015-0672-x

[12] Edwards TA, Daly C, Donovan RL, Whitehouse MR. Risk of complications following surgical fixation of femoral diaphyseal fractures in children aged 4 to 12 years: A systematic review and meta-analysis. Injury. 2022;**53**:1020–1028. DOI: 10.1016/j.injury.2021.11.005

[13] Böstman O, Pihlajamäki H. Clinical biocompatibility of biodegradable orthopaedic implants for internal fixation: A review. Biomaterials. 2000;**21**:2615–2621. DOI: 10.1016/s0142-9612(00)00129-0

[14] Aikin M, Shalomeev V, Kukhar V, Kostryzhev A, Kuziev I, Kulynych V, et al. Recent advances in biodegradable magnesium alloys for medical implants: Evolution, innovations, and clinical translation. Crystals. Multidisciplinary Digital Publishing Institute. 2025;**15**:671

[15] Brar H, Platt M, Sarntinoranont M, Martin P, Manuel M. Magnesium as a biodegradable and bioabsorbable material for medical Implants. JOM: Journal of the Minerals, Metals & Materials Society. 2009;**61**:31–34. DOI: 10.1007/s11837-009-0129-0

[16] Böstman O, Hirvensalo E, Vainionpää S, Mäkelä A, Vihtonen K, Törmälä P, et al. Ankle fractures treated using biodegradable internal fixation. Clinical Orthopaedics and Related Research. 1989;**238**:195–203

[17] Hope PG, Williamson DM, Coates CJ, Cole WG. Biodegradable pin fixation of elbow fractures in children. A randomised trial. The Journal of Bone and Joint Surgery. British Volume. 1991;**73**:965–968. DOI: 10.1302/0301-620X.73B6.1659570

[18] Svensson PJ, Janarv PM, Hirsch G. Internal fixation with biodegradable rods in pediatric fractures: One-year follow-up of fifty patients. Journal of Pediatric Orthopaedics. 1994;**14**:220–224. DOI: 10.1097/01241398-199403000-00017

[19] Böstman OM, Pihlajamäki HK. Adverse tissue reactions to bioabsorbable fixation devices. Clinical Orthopaedics and Related Research. 2000;**371**:216–227

[20] Elmowafy EM, Tiboni M, Soliman ME. Biocompatibility, biodegradation and biomedical applications of poly(lactic acid)/poly (lactic-co-glycolic acid) micro and nanoparticles. Journal of Pharmaceutical Investigation. 2019;**49**:347–380. DOI: 10.1007/s40005-019-00439-x

[21] Kovacevic S, Ali W, Mandal TK, Martínez-Pañeda E, LLorca J. Impact of pH and chloride content on the biodegradation of magnesium alloys for medical implants: An in vitro and phase-field study. Acta Biomaterialia. 2025;**198**:546–565. DOI: 10.1016/j.actbio.2025.03.034

[22] Perhomaa M, Pokka T, Korhonen L, Kyrö A, Niinimäki J, Serlo W, et al. Randomized controlled trial of the clinical recovery and biodegradation of polylactide-co-glycolide implants used in the intramedullary nailing of children's forearm shaft fractures with at least four years of follow-up. Journal of Clinical Medicine. 2021;**10**:995

[23] Das S, Seesala VS, Basu B, Mukherjee S. PLGA-based resorbable implants for biomedical applications: Manufacturing, biocompatibility, and clinical translation. Materials Today Communications. 2025;**49**:114116. DOI: 10.1016/j.mtcomm.2025.114116

[24] Gentile P, Chiono V, Carmagnola I, Hatton PV. An overview of poly (lactic-co-glycolic) acid (PLGA)-based biomaterials for bone tissue engineering. International Journal of Molecular Sciences. 2014;**15**:3640–3659. DOI: 10.3390/ijms15033640

[25] Bostman O, Hirvensalo E, Makinen J, Rokkanen P. Foreign-body reactions to fracture fixation implants of biodegradable synthetic polymers. The Journal of Bone and Joint Surgery. British Volume. 1990;**72-B**:592–596. DOI: 10.1302/0301-620X.72B4.2199452

[26] Lu Y, Zhang T, Chen K, Canavese F, Huang C, Yang H, et al. Application of biodegradable implants in pediatric orthopedics: Shifting from absorbable polymers to biodegradable metals. Bioactive Materials. 2025;**50**:189–214

[27] Sheikh Z, Najeeb S, Khurshid Z, Verma V, Rashid H, Glogauer M. Biodegradable materials for bone repair and tissue engineering applications. Materials (Basel, Switzerland). 2015;**8**:5744–5794. DOI: 10.3390/ma8095273

[28] Sabir MI, Xu X, Li L. A review on biodegradable polymeric materials for bone tissue engineering applications. Journal of Materials Science. 2009;**44**:5713–5724. DOI: 10.1007/s10853-009-3770-7

[29] Landes CA, Ballon A, Roth C. In-patient versus in vitro degradation of P(L/DL)LA and PLGA. Journal of Biomedical Materials Research Part B: Applied Biomaterials. 2006;**76**:403–411. DOI: 10.1002/jbm.b.30388

[30] Eastwood F, Raheman F, Al-Dairy G, Popescu M, Henney C, Hunwick L, et al. Healing smarter: A systematic review and meta-analysis of bioresorbable implants for paediatric forearm fractures. Journal of Children's Orthopaedics. 2025;**19**:422–431

[31] Gareb B, van Bakelen NB, Dijkstra PU, Vissink A, Bos RRM, van Minnen B. Biodegradable versus titanium osteosynthesis in maxillofacial traumatology: A systematic review with meta-analysis and trial sequential analysis. International Journal of Oral and Maxillofacial Surgery. 2020;**49**:914–931. DOI: 10.1016/j.ijom.2019.11.009

[32] Rocha CV, Gonçalves V, da Silva MC, Bañobre-López M, Gallo J. PLGA-Based Composites for Various Biomedical Applications. International Journal of Molecular Sciences. 2022;**23**:2034. DOI: 10.3390/ijms23042034

[33] Barber FA, Spenciner DB, Bhattacharyya S, Miller LE. Biocomposite Implants Composed of Poly(Lactide-co-Glycolide)/β-Tricalcium Phosphate: Systematic Review of Imaging, Complication, and Performance Outcomes. Arthroscopy: The Journal of Arthroscopic & Related Surgery. 2017;**33**:683–689. DOI: 10.1016/j.arthro.2016.09.032

[34] Baldini M, Coppa V, Falcioni D, Senigagliesi E, Marinelli M, Gigante AP. Use of resorbable magnesium screws in children: Systematic review of the literature and short-term follow-up from our series. Journal of Children's Orthopaedics. 2022;**16**:77–80. DOI: 10.1177/18632521221080032

[35] Schlechter JA, Nguyen SV, Fletcher KL. Utility of bioabsorbable fixation of osteochondral lesions in the adolescent knee: Outcomes analysis with minimum 2-year follow-up. Orthopaedic Journal of Sports Medicine. 2019;7:2325967119876896. DOI: 10.1177/2325967119876896

[36] Kim WS, Oh MJ, Park MS, Sung KH. Comparison of surgical outcomes between bioabsorbable and metal screw fixation for distal tibial physeal fracture in children and adolescent. International Orthopaedics. 2024;**48**:2681–2687. DOI: 10.1007/s00264-024-06284-4

[37] Liu J, Pathak G, Joshi M, Andrews K, Lee J. A meta-analysis comparing the outcomes of syndesmotic

injury treated with metal screw, dynamic fixation, and bioabsorbable screw. Journal of Orthopaedics. 2021;**25**:82–87. DOI: 10.1016/j.jor.2021.04.006

[38] Chen T, Wen Y, Zhu D, Feng W, Song B, Wang Q. Comparison of bioabsorbable screw versus metallic screw fixation for tibial tubercle fractures in adolescents: A retrospective cohort study. BMC Musculoskeletal Disorders. 2025;**26**:38. DOI: 10.1186/s12891-025-08281-z

[39] Tóth Z, Kassai T, Varga M, Molnár T, Antal E, Lamberti AG, et al. Treatment of pediatric displaced intraarticular olecranon fractures with resorbable Poly-L-Lactic-Co-Glycolic Acid (PLGA) Pins and Polydioxanone (PDS) loops. Children. 2025;**12**:316

[40] Korhonen L, Perhomaa M, Kyrö A, Pokka T, Serlo W, Merikanto J, et al. Intramedullary nailing of forearm shaft fractures by biodegradable compared with titanium nails: Results of a prospective randomized trial in children with at least two years of follow-up. Biomaterials. 2018;**185**: 383–392

[41] Gkiokas A, Morassi LG, Kohl S, Zampakides C, Megremis P, Evangelopoulos DS. Bioabsorbable pins for treatment of osteochondral fractures of the knee after acute patella dislocation in children and young adolescents. Advances in Orthopedics. 2012;2012e249687. DOI: 10.1155/2012/249687

[42] Baldini M, Coppa V, Falcioni D, Cusano G, Massetti D, Marinelli M, et al. Resorbable magnesium screws for fixation of medial epicondyle avulsion fractures in skeletally immature patients: A comparison with Kirschner wires. Journal of Children's Orthopaedics. 2022;**16**:481–487

[43] Rafi BM, Tiwari V. Forearm Fractures. StatPearls [Internet]. Treasure Island (FL): StatPearls Publishing; 2025, November 15. Available from: https://www.ncbi.nlm.nih.gov/books/NBK574580/ [Accessed: 2025-November-15]

[44] Caruso G, Caldari E, Sturla FD, Caldaria A, Re DL, Pagetti P, et al. Management of pediatric forearm fractures: What is the best therapeutic choice? A narrative review of the literature. Musculoskeletal SURGERY. 2021;**105**:225–234

[45] Roeder C, Alves C, Balslev-Clausen A, Canavese F, Gercek E, Kassai T, et al. Pilot study and preliminary results of biodegradable intramedullary nailing of forearm fractures in children. Child Basel Switz. 2022;**9**:754

[46] Hedelin H, Hebelka H, Brisby H, Laine T. MRI evaluation of resorbable poly lactic-co-glycolic acid (PLGA) screws used in pelvic osteotomies in children—a retrospective case series. Journal of Orthopaedic Surgery and Research. 2020;**15**:329. DOI: 10.1186/s13018-020-01858-5

[47] da Costa AP, Rodrigues ET, Hauache HA, Fujisaki MA, Dobashi ET. Comparative analysis of treatments for forearm fractures in children: A systematic review and meta-analysis. Acta Ortop Bras. 2025;33e290231. DOI: 10.1590/1413-785220253306e290231

[48] Clavicle Fractures - Midshaft - Trauma - Orthobullets [Internet]. 2025, November 15. Available from: https://www.orthobullets.com/trauma/1011/cl

avicle-fractures–midshaft?hideLeftMenu=true [Accessed: 2025-November-15]

[49] Osborn EJ, Farnsworth CL, Doan JD, Edmonds EW. Bioabsorbable plating in the treatment of pediatric clavicle fractures: A biomechanical and clinical analysis. Clinical Biomechanics. 2018;**55**:94–99. DOI: 10.1016/j.clinbiomech.2018.04.017

[50] Markes AR, Garcia-Lopez E, Halvorson RT, Swarup I. Management of displaced midshaft clavicle fractures in pediatrics and adolescents: Operative vs nonoperative treatment. Orthopedic Research and Reviews. 2022;**14**:373–381. DOI: 10.2147/ORR.S340538

[51] Lim JA, Loh BL, Sylvestor G, Khan W. Perioperative management of distal radius fractures. Journal of Perioperative Practice. 2021;**31**:1750458920949463. DOI: 10.1177/1750458920949463

[52] Ilyas AM. Surgical approaches to the distal radius. Hand (New York, N.Y.). 2011;**6**:8–17. DOI: 10.1007/s11552-010-9281-9

[53] Olech J, Ciszewski M, Morasiewicz P. Epidemiology of distal radius fractures in children and adults during the COVID-19 pandemic – A two-center study. BMC Musculoskeletal Disorders. 2021;**22**:306. DOI: 10.1186/s12891-021-04128-5

[54] Distal Radius Fractures - Trauma - Orthobullets [Internet]. 2025, November 15. Available from: https://www.orthobullets.com/trauma/1027/distal-radius-fractures?hideLeftMenu=true [Accessed: 2025-November-15]

[55] Seigerman D, Lutsky K, Fletcher D, Katt B, Kwok M, Mazur D, et al. Complications in the Management of Distal Radius fractures: How do we avoid them? Current Reviews in Musculoskeletal Medicine. 2019;**12**: 204–212

[56] Chung KC, Mathews AL. Management of complications of distal radius fractures. Hand Clinics. 2015;**31**:205–215. DOI: 10.1016/j.hcl.2014.12.002

[57] Varga M, Józsa G, Hanna D, Tóth M, Hajnal B, Krupa Z, et al. Bioresorbable implants vs. Kirschner-wires in the treatment of severely displaced distal paediatric radius and forearm fractures - a retrospective multicentre study. BMC Musculoskeletal Disorders. 2022;**23**:362

[58] Klahs KJ, Dertinger JE, Mello GT, Thapa K, Sandler AB, Garcia EJJ, et al. Epidemiologic investigation of pediatric distal humerus fractures: An American insurance claims database study. World Journal of Orthopedics. 2024;**15**:52–60

[59] Martins T, Tiwari V, Marappa-Ganeshan R Pediatric Lateral Humeral Condyle Fractures. StatPearls [Internet]. Treasure Island (FL): StatPearls Publishing; 2025, November 16. Available from: https://www.ncbi.nlm.nih.gov/books/NBK560664/ [Accessed: 2025-November-16]

[60] Schroeder K, Gilbert S, Ellington M, Souder C, Yang S. Pediatric lateral humeral condyle fractures: Current concept review. Journal of the Pediatric Orthopaedic Society of North America. 2020;**2**:82. DOI: 10.55275/JPOSNA-2020-82

[61] Stelmach W, Beczkowski J, Zając P, Małecki K, Sibiński M, Niedzielski K. Clinical and radiological evaluation of surgical treatment of medial epicondyle

fractures of humerus in children. A two-centre study. Scientific Reports. 2023;**13**:10095. DOI: 10.1038/s41598-023-37063-7

[62] Hahn SG, Schuller A, Pichler L, Hohensteiner A, Sator T, Bamer O, et al. Complications and outcomes of surgically treated pediatric supracondylar humerus fractures. Children. Multidisciplinary Digital Publishing Institute. 2024;**11**:791

[63] Del Valle-Hernández E, Marrero-Barrera PA, Beaton D, Bravo D, Santiago S, Guzmán-Pérez H, et al. Complications associated with pediatric supracondylar humeral fractures. Puerto Rico Health Sciences Journal. 2017;**36**:37–40

[64] Zeng M, Xie K, Cao S, Wen J, Wang S, Xiao S. Midterm comparative result of absorbable screws and metal screws in pediatric medial humeral epicondyle fracture. Journal of Orthopaedic Science. 2025;**30**:824–829. DOI: 10.1016/j.jos.2024.12.004

[65] Sinikumpu -J-J, Serlo W. Biodegradable poly-L-lactide-co-glycolide copolymer pin fixation of a traumatic patellar osteochondral fragment in an 11-year-old child: A novel surgical approach. Experimental and Therapeutic Medicine. 2017;**13**:242–246. DOI: 10.3892/etm.2016.3934

[66] Perkins CA, Busch MT, Christino MA, Axelrod J, Devito DP, Fabregas JA, et al. Olecranon fractures in children and adolescents: Outcomes based on fracture fixation. Journal of Children's Orthopaedics. 2018;**12**: 497–501

[67] De Maio F, Gorgolini G, Caterini A, Luciano C, Covino D, Farsetti P. Treatment of olecranon fractures in childhood: A systematic review. Frontiers in Pediatrics. 2022;**10**:1046243. DOI: 10.3389/fped.2022.1046243

[68] Holme TJ, Karbowiak M, Arnander M, Gelfer Y. Paediatric olecranon fractures: A systematic review. EFORT Open Reviews. 2020;**5**:280–288. DOI: 10.1302/2058-5241.5.190082

[69] Bauer KL. Osteochondral injuries of the knee in pediatric patients. The Journal of Knee Surgery. 2018;**31**:382–391. DOI: 10.1055/s-0038-1625956

[70] Pechlivanidou E, Zambakides C, Margariti RE. Pediatric osteochondral fractures: Clinical insights associate early diagnosis to early rehabilitation via arthroscopy. European Journal of Orthopaedic Surgery & Traumatology. 2024;**34**:1657–1665. DOI: 10.1007/s00590-024-03852-7

[71] Walsh SJ, Boyle MJ, Morganti V. Large osteochondral fractures of the lateral femoral condyle in the adolescent: Outcome of bioabsorbable pin fixation. The Journal of Bone and Joint Surgery-American Volume. 2008;**90**:1473–1478. DOI: 10.2106/JBJS.G.00595

[72] Hollander JJ, Dahmen J, Emanuel KS, Stufkens SAS, Kennedy JG, Kerkhoffs GMMJ. The frequency and severity of complications in surgical treatment of osteochondral lesions of the talus: A systematic review and meta-analysis of 6,962 lesions. Cartilage. 2023;**14**:180–197. DOI: 10.1177/19476035231154746

[73] Kühle J, Angele P, Balcarek P, Eichinger M, Feucht M, Haasper C, et al. Treatment of osteochondral fractures of

the knee: A meta-analysis of available scientific evidence. International Orthopaedics. 2013;**37**:2385–2394

[74] Felus J, Kowalczyk B, Starmach M, Wyrobek L. Osteochondral fractures in acute patellar dislocations in adolescents: Midterm results of surgical treatment. Orthopaedic Journal of Sports Medicine. 2022;**10**:23259671221107608. DOI: 10.1177/23259671221107608

[75] Khan SA, Baghdadi S, Carey JL, Moores TS, Sheth NP, Ganley T. Osteochondral fractures after patellar dislocation: Current concepts. JAAOS Global Research and Reviews. 2021;5e2100155. DOI: 10.5435/JAAOSGlobal-D-21-00155

[76] Weber CD, Migliorini F, Hildebrand F. Reconstruction of large osteochondral lesions in the knee: Focus on fixation techniques. Life. Multidisciplinary Digital Publishing Institute. 2021;**11**:543. DOI: 10.3390/life11060543

[77] Małecki K, Pruchnik–Witosławska K, Gwizdała D, Grzelak P, Flont P, Niedzielski KR. Clinical results and MRI evaluation of patellar osteochondral fracture fixation following patellar dislocation. BioMed Research International. 2019;**2019**:7943636. DOI: 10.1155/2019/7943636

[78] Podeszwa DA, Wilson PL, Holland AR, Copley LAB. Comparison of bioabsorbable versus metallic implant fixation for physeal and epiphyseal fractures of the distal tibia. Journal of Pediatric Orthopaedics. 2008;**28**: 859–863. DOI: 10.1097/BPO.0b013e31818e19d7

[79] Noh JH, Roh YH, Yang BG, Kim SW, Lee JS, Oh MK. Outcomes of operative treatment of unstable ankle fractures: A comparison of metallic and biodegradable implants. The Journal of Bone and Joint Surgery-American Volume. 2012;94e166. DOI: 10.2106/JBJS.K.01221

[80] Nudelman H, Lőrincz A, Lamberti AG, Varga M, Kassai T, Józsa G. Management of pediatric ankle fractures: Comparison of biodegradable PLGA implants with traditional metal screws. Frontiers in Pediatrics. 2024;**12**:1410750. DOI: 10.3389/fped.2024.1410750

[81] Li Z-H, Yu A-X, Guo X-P, Qi B-W, Zhou M, Wang W-Y. Absorbable implants versus metal implants for the treatment of ankle fractures: A meta-analysis. Experimental and Therapeutic Medicine. 2013;**5**:1531–1537. DOI: 10.3892/etm.2013.1017

[82] Egerci OF, Dogruoz F, Cetin H, Ertan MB, Yapar A, Kose O. High rate of failure after magnesium bioabsorbable compression screw fixation for scaphoid fractures. Journal of Orthopaedic Surgery and Research. 2025;**20**:296. DOI: 10.1186/s13018-025-05701-7

[83] Könneker S, Schächinger U, Vogt PM. Magnesium-based compression screws in acute scaphoid fractures and nonunions. World Journal of Surgery. 2023;**47**:1129–1135. DOI: 10.1007/s00268-023-06937-2

[84] Polat O, Toy S, Kibar B. Surgical outcomes of scaphoid fracture osteosynthesis with magnesium screws. Joint Diseases and Related Surgery. 2021;**32**:721–728. DOI: 10.52312/jdrs.2021.298

[85] Blackman B, Okunbor S, Sowa AM, McDonnell JM, Ross TD, Rigney B, et al. Bioabsorbable implants are a viable alternative to traditional metallic

implants in orthopaedic surgery: A systematic review and meta-analysis. Journal of Orthopaedics. 2025;**65**: 257–269

[86] Kitridis D, Savvidis P, Cheva A, Papalois A, Givissis P, Chalidis B. Are absorbable plates more resistant to infection than titanium implants? An experimental pre-clinical trial in rabbits. Journal of Functional Biomaterials. 2023;**14**:498. DOI: 10.3390/jfb14100498

[87] Müller E, Schoberwalter T, Mader K, Seitz J-M, Kopp A, Baranowsky A, et al. The biological effects of magnesium-based implants on the skeleton and their clinical implications in orthopedic trauma surgery. Biomaterials Research. 2024;**28**:0122

[88] Yang Y, Zhou X, Zhang M, Zhou Y, Wang B, Yuan C. Lateral wall osteotomy combined with embedded biodegradable implants for displaced intra-articular calcaneal fractures. Journal of Orthopaedic Surgery and Research. 2019;**14**:74. DOI: 10.1186/s13018-019-1111-3

[89] Sabir MI, Xu X, Li L. (PDF) A review on biodegradable polymeric materials for bone tissue engineering applications. Journal of Materials Science. 2025;**44**:5713–5724. DOI: 10.1007/s10853-009-3770-7

[90] Hedelin H, Larnert P, Antonsson P, Lagerstrand K, Brisby H, Hebelka H, et al. Stability in pelvic triple osteotomies in children using resorbable PLGA screws for fixation. Journal of Pediatric Orthopaedics. 2021:41e787. DOI: 10.1097/BPO.0000000000001873

[91] Hung CH, Kwok YC, Yip J, Wong HH, Leung YY. Bioabsorbable magnesium-based materials potential and safety in bone surgery: A systematic review. Craniomaxillofacial Trauma & Reconstruction. 2025;**18**:24. DOI: 10.3390/cmtr18020024

[92] Bioretec. CE mark approval for remeos^{tm} trauma screw product group, featuring four product lines with over 200 individual products, drives global expansion for bioretec [Internet]. 2025, November 16. Available from: https://www.prnewswire.com/news-releases/ce-mark-approval-for-remeos-trauma-screw-product-group-featuring-four-product-lines-with-over-200-individual-products-drives-global-expansion-for-bioretec-302377207.html [Accessed: 2025-November-16]

Chapter 2

Innovative Orthopedics in Serbia: Personalized Orthopedic Treatment Using Computer-Aided Design and Manufacturing

Milutin Micic, Branislav Krivokapic and Jelena Jadzic

Abstract

Personalized therapeutic approaches to treating orthopedic conditions involve adapting treatment protocols to the unique anatomical characteristics, medical history, and patient needs (i.e., lifestyle, habits, and personal goals). Modern studies emphasize that computer-aided design (CAD) and computer-aided manufacturing (CAM) improve orthopedic treatment outcomes, shorten surgical time, reduce the risk of complications, and consequently lower costs to the healthcare system. In our country, specific challenges of an innovative orthopedic approach include the development of personalized 3D-printed medical models for alloarthroplasty, the use of virtual surgical planning, the development of personalized 3D models for planning complex orthopedic surgeries, the creation of personalized surgical guides for the resection of bone tumors, and the adequate restoration of resulting bone defects. This chapter aims to provide an insight into our novel research activities regarding the use of 3D printing in orthopedics in Serbia, following two main research directions. The first direction of our research involves improving the quality of 3D reconstructions of radiological images obtained using various protocols/methods, with the aim of enhancing the outcomes of computer-assisted surgery (CAS), virtual surgical planning, and the production of personalized surgical guides and medical models. The second direction of our research involves the use of tissue engineering methods in orthopedics (i.e., selection of appropriate bone substitutes, design of tissue scaffolds, and modeling of personalized orthopedic implants and orthoses). In this chapter, we aim to highlight our recent research on the clinical potential of personalized 3D-printed orthoses for patients with distal radius fractures to promote accelerated bone fracture healing.

Keywords: orthopedics, computer-guided surgery, virtual surgical planning, 3D printing, tissue engineering

1. Introduction

The use of 3D printing in biomedicine is primarily related to the concept of personalized medicine, i.e., effectively planning, designing, and conducting

IntechOpen

patient-specific medical treatments [1]. About 90% of the total use of 3D printing in medicine is in surgery, with the most dominant fields of 3D printing implementation being in knee and maxillofacial surgery [2, 3]. The use of innovative approaches in personalized skeletal reconstructions follows two complementary research directions. The first research direction consists of bone substitutes (bone replacement materials) engineering and cellular and acellular bone scaffold production, with the potential to be used during orthopedic surgeries [4–6]. Still, the participation of this research approach in the overall use of 3D printing for skeletal reconstruction remains relatively low due to several reasons. Firstly, the complexity of the hierarchical organization of bone tissue [7] should be mimicked with bone replacement materials to ensure osteointegration (incorporation into surrounding bone), osteoconduction (facilitating nutrient transport), and osteoinduction (inducing new bone formation) of the generated implant [8]. Further, these morphological assessments should be integrated with computational models, which should include the dynamic change of the mechanobiological environment [9]. Additionally, the specific and complex requirements for adapting 3D printing technology to the production of such implants are challenging, even with modern technology [10, 11]. Furthermore, the majority of these research approaches are still in the early phase (proof-of-concept and animal research) [11]. Although the potential of animal model research should not be overlooked, this chapter is primarily focused on innovative orthopedic approaches in human studies.

The second research direction encompasses the entire clinical process, from initial patient management and radiological diagnostics to therapy planning, utilizing computer-aided design (CAD) and computer-aided manufacturing (CAM) for the creation of medical models and surgical guides [12–15]. Contemporary studies have demonstrated that the use of medical models and surgical guides is associated with a significant reduction in surgery time, a decrease in ischemia time, and a reduction in postoperative risks, while also providing a more predictable outcome and lower treatment costs [16–19]. Still, despite a plethora of scientific publications, the clinical application of 3D printing in orthopedics remains very limited compared to its demands, especially in low- to middle-income countries [19–21]. One of the leading reasons is a mismatch between the medical and engineering chain-link, usually because the production facilities (with 3D printers and other necessary equipment) are distant from the clinic where the patient is being treated. Moreover, preoperative CAD/CAM procedures require considerable involvement of the orthopedic surgeon, who is often not a part of the virtual planning and 3D printing teams [12]. The issue is further complicated by the time-pressing requirement of the disease being treated to avoid inadequate healing and other complications that may affect treatment outcomes. Lastly, the lack of standardized procedures and associated costs are limiting the generalizability of the clinical application of 3D printing in orthopedics.

This chapter aims to introduce the reader to the varieties and achievements of 3D printing in skeletal reconstruction, to explain the specific challenges and potential directions for future research involving the use of 3D printing in orthopedics, and to describe the concrete results of this innovative orthopedic approach in Serbia, with special emphasis on highlighting certain advantages and disadvantages of available 3D printing technologies in medicine.

2. CAD/CAM in orthopedics: Our and global research experience

The advent of personalized orthopedic treatments has revolutionized the field of musculoskeletal medicine, addressing the inherent limitations of one-size-fits-all approaches that often fail to account for individual anatomical variations, biomechanical needs, and pathological specificities, thereby underscoring the critical necessity for CAD/CAM technologies to enhance precision, efficacy, and patient outcomes [20]. Traditional orthopedic interventions, such as off-the-shelf implants and standardized surgical procedures, frequently result in suboptimal fits, increased revision rates, and prolonged recovery times due to mismatches between generic devices and the unique geometries of patients' bones, joints, and soft tissues – problems that CAD/CAM systems mitigate by enabling the creation of bespoke solutions tailored to each individual's morphology. This approach allows clinicians to digitize patient data from imaging modalities like computed tomography (CT) scans, magnetic resonance imaging (MRI), and 3D surface scans, generating virtual models that simulate anatomical structures with millimeter-level accuracy (**Figure 1**), which in turn facilitates the design of custom implants, prosthetics, and surgical guides that align perfectly with the patient's body, reducing intraoperative complications and postoperative discomfort [20, 22]. This personalization is particularly important in complex cases such as joint replacements for patients with

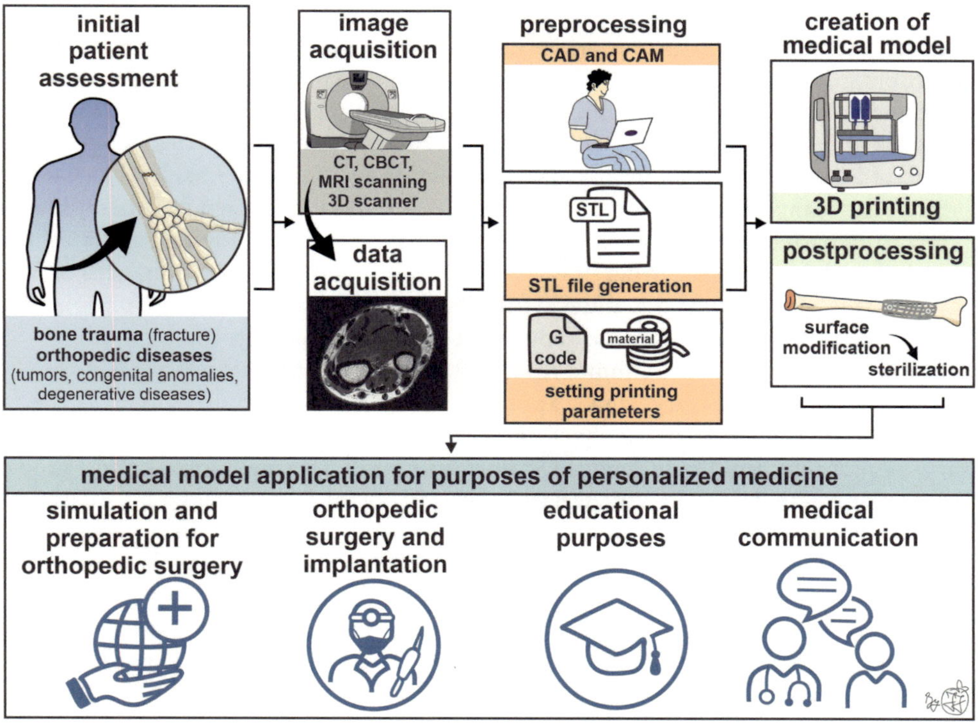

Figure 1.
Schematic representation of the step-by-step approach to the use of 3D printing in orthopedics. Abbreviations: CT – computed tomography; CBCT – cone beam computed tomography; MRI – magnetic resonance imaging; CAD – computer-aided design; CAM – computer-aided manufacturing.

congenital deformities, traumatic injuries, or degenerative conditions like osteoarthritis, where standard implants may lead to instability, wear, or failure. Our initial research was focused on the use of 3D printing in the tertiary maxillofacial clinic in Serbia to facilitate mandibular reconstruction surgeries [23]. We tested eight different scanning protocols used for the precise 3D printing of mandibular models and assessed linear measures on the human mandible, comparing them with CT/CBCT digital scans and 3D-printed medical models of the mandible [23]. Our research distinguished that a specific CT protocol could serve as a single radiologic protocol used to scan both donor and recipient regions during the preoperative phase of mandibular reconstruction [23]. A large scanning field of view obtained with the CT scanning protocol is valuable in patients requiring mandibular reconstruction, as it enables assessing the surrounding regions for possible secondary injuries or tumors. Since measurement misalignments could lead to problems with surgical guides and reconstruction grafts for bone tissue, we provided practical guidelines for correcting the 3D reconstructions and their physical 3D-printed mandibular models to improve the outcome of reconstructive procedures in maxillofacial surgery [23].

Furthermore, CAD/CAM empowers orthopedic surgeons to iterate designs virtually, optimizing factors such as load distribution, material properties, and integration with surrounding tissues before physical production (**Figure 1**). CAM processes translate these digital blueprints into tangible devices using biocompatible materials, such as titanium alloys or polymers, ensuring rapid prototyping and production that can be completed in days rather than weeks. This expedites treatment timelines and improves accessibility in resource-limited settings. The need for such technologies is further amplified by the growing prevalence of bone health disorders in aging populations, where personalized treatments can significantly lower healthcare costs by minimizing revisions. Previous studies have shown that custom CAD/CAM implants can reduce the need for revision surgeries by up to 30% compared to conventional methods, as they better accommodate skeletal variations [15]. In the realm of reconstructive surgery, CAD/CAM has proven indispensable for fabricating patient-specific titanium meshes for alveolar bone augmentation in maxillofacial orthopedics, where precise contouring to defect sites enhances bone regeneration and esthetic outcomes, with deviations as low as 0.5 mm from planned models [24]. Recently, our group reported a novel clinical protocol for total maxillectomy with pterygoid bone resection and consecutive microvascular reconstruction using a harvested scapula tip flap [25]. This protocol involves the immediate placement of extra-short implants in donor bone, facilitated by virtual surgical planning and the *in-house* 3D printing of medical models and surgical guides in a tertiary maxillofacial clinic in Serbia [25]. In spinal orthopedics, CAD/CAM systems enable the design of customized cervical orthoses that conform to the patient's neck curvature, providing superior immobilization and comfort over generic braces, which often cause pressure sores or inadequate support [26, 27]. Recent advancements in CAD/CAM have enabled the incorporation of lightweight, breathable materials produced via selective laser sintering, thereby enhancing patient compliance and functional recovery [13].

Beyond implants and orthotics, the integration of CAD/CAM in surgical planning through computer-assisted surgery (CAS) systems allows for preoperative simulations that predict orthopedic outcomes, refine incision placements, and guide instrumentation (**Figure 1**), thereby reducing operative time and minimizing blood loss, which is crucial in high-risk procedures like total hip arthroplasty or tumor resections [14]. This predictive capability is bolstered by the synergy with emerging technologies such as digital twins, virtual replicas of patients' anatomies that simulate physiological responses to interventions, offering orthopedic surgeons a tool to anticipate complications in non-union fractures and plan revisions with unprecedented accuracy, potentially decreasing failure rates in complex trauma cases [28]. Furthermore, CAD/CAM facilitates multidisciplinary collaboration, allowing surgeons, engineers, prosthetists, and physiatrists to co-design solutions in real-time via cloud-based platforms, which is essential for addressing the diverse needs of patients with amputations, where custom prosthetic sockets designed through CAD scanning ensure better socket-limb interfaces, reducing skin breakdowns and improving gait efficiency [29].

The economic imperative for CAD/CAM in personalized orthopedics is not to be overlooked. By streamlining manufacturing processes, these technologies reduce material waste and production costs, making high-quality, tailored treatments more viable for widespread adoption, especially in developing countries where access to specialized care is limited. Experimental studies on CAD simulations in complex orthopedic procedures have highlighted their safety, user-friendliness, and cost-effectiveness, with tools like patient-specific instrumentation improving alignment accuracy in knee replacements, leading to better long-term joint function and reduced wear on prostheses [30]. Advances in 3D printing, closely tied to CAD/CAM workflows, have expanded applications to include bioresorbable scaffolds for bone defects, where custom designs promote tissue ingrowth and natural healing, as evidenced by recent developments showing enhanced surgical efficiency and accuracy [1]. Our colleagues from the University of Nis have pioneered methods for human bone redesign using Non-Uniform Rational Catmull-Clark Surfaces with T-junctions in CAD environments, offering superior efficiency over traditional Non-Uniform Rational B-Splines for modeling complex topologies in personalized endoprostheses and biodegradable scaffolds, as demonstrated in mandibular reconstructions of congenital defects, underscoring how such innovations can streamline surgical planning and manufacturing in resource-constrained Serbian settings [31]. Similarly, collaborative efforts involving Serbian academics from the University of Belgrade integrate CAD/CAM with rapid prototyping for long bone orthopedics, employing finite element analysis to simulate walking kinematics and optimize implant designs, which is crucial for addressing prevalent conditions like osteoarthritis and fractures in a population facing healthcare strains from underfunding and equipment obsolescence [32]. Thus, CAD/CAM not only bridges anatomical individuality with therapeutic efficacy but also helps position a hub for innovative, cost-effective personalized orthopedics, ensuring better functional restoration and quality of life for patients navigating systemic challenges in Serbia.

3. The role of 3D printing in orthopedics in Serbia

According to the official report from the Statistical Office of the Republic of Serbia, approximately 23% of Serbia's population is older than 65 years [33], which is a higher percentage than the EU average [34]. An increasing percentage of the elderly population is burdening the public health system with geriatric diseases, among which the most taxing are osteoporosis and bone fractures that do not heal adequately, non-union fractures due to metabolic problems, and problems with mobility in elderly people. Available data on the Serbian public healthcare system for the 2005–2019 period [35] show that the number of new cases of cancer rose from 24,755 to 41,661, the number of hospital discharges for all cancers doubled, hospital discharges for ischemic heart disease went from 36,432 to 53,112, hospital discharges for musculoskeletal system and connective tissue diseases went from 54,505 to 81,844, the number of all hospital discharges increased by around 17%, while the number of hospitals and physicians working in hospitals stayed roughly the same. During the COVID-19 pandemic, the situation in the Serbian healthcare system became increasingly complicated, with a focus on the pressing issue of immunization, where the main investments and improvements were made. Having all this in mind, it is understandable that CAD-CAM or 3D printing in orthopedics was not a priority for a resource-limited healthcare system in Serbia, but rather a matter of initiative by small bone research teams [33]. A recent exception is the ongoing GovTech program of the Innovation Fund of the Republic of Serbia, where we are conducting a clinical study about the use of 3D-printed personalized orthoses in the treatment of distal forearm fractures, along with training and development of the CAD-CAM team for complicated orthopedic surgeries.

In our country, specific challenges of an innovative orthopedic approach include the development of personalized 3D-printed medical models for alloarthroplasty, the use of virtual surgical planning, the development of personalized 3D models for planning complex orthopedic surgeries, the creation of personalized surgical guides for the resection of bone tumors, and the adequate restoration of the resulting bone defects. This chapter aims to provide insight into our novel research activities regarding the use of 3D printing in orthopedics in Serbia. The first direction of our research involves improving the quality of 3D reconstructions of radiological images obtained using various radiological protocols, with the aim of enhancing the surgical outcomes. We have successfully demonstrated that the implementation of virtual surgery planning and *in-house* 3D-printed surgical guides resulted in a reduction of total surgery time by 1.4 hours, with a significant reduction in average hospitalization time, while significantly increasing final functional and esthetic results, as well as patient satisfaction [33]. The second direction of our research involves the use of tissue engineering methods in orthopedics (i.e., selection of adequate bone substitutes, design of tissue scaffolds, and modeling of personalized orthopedic implants). Aligned with this, we developed and prototyped an acellular 3D bioprinter for bone scaffold fabrication [11] using a novel bone replacement material made of nanohydroxyapatite with a poly(lactide-co-glycolide) coating. The mentioned bone replacement material (ALBO-OS) is currently under finalization of a clinical trial, while our 3D bioprinter for bone scaffold fabrication has been verified only in an animal model [11]. Further, we focused our research interest on the clinical potential of using personalized 3D-printed orthoses in patients with distal radius fractures to promote accelerated bone fracture healing. The overall goal of both research directions within our team is to make methods for virtual surgical planning and *in-house* 3D printing of patient-specific instrumentation available and to standardize their use in Serbia. Furthermore, the role of orthopedic surgeons as prescribers of these technologies is evolving, requiring them to engage actively in the design process to ensure clinical relevance, as passive adoption may overlook nuanced anatomical considerations [12]. In orthotic fabrication, CAD/CAM systems, like those used in physical medicine and rehabilitation departments, provide state-of -the-art tools for precise fitting, addressing conditions such as foot deformities or post-stroke hemiplegia with devices that adapt to dynamic movements [36]. These data highlight the need for high-quality education for Serbian orthopedic surgeons/physiatrists to facilitate the integration of 3D printing into our healthcare system. An interesting application of 3D printing in orthopedics could be in obtaining accurate human anatomy models (**Figure 1**), which can be used to facilitate the education of medical students and young clinicians in Serbia [37].

4. Clinical potential of using personalized 3D-printed orthoses in patients with bone fractures: Current limitations and future directions

3D printing of personalized orthoses is an interesting subfield that deals with CAD-CAM in orthopedics [38]. Since distal radius fractures are the most common [28], this emerging subfield is almost exclusively dedicated to this type of fracture. Minor limitations of traditional forearm plaster casts or synthetic orthoses used for distal radius fracture treatment include that patients reporting that the cast is heavy and uncomfortable, it impairs personal hygiene, and can cause skin irritation [39]. Additionally, if inadequately placed and shaped, it can cause nerve dysfunction [40, 41]. A major limitation is the risk of secondary dislocation, which can occur in more than 70% of cases, particularly in the elderly population [42]. Initial swelling at the fracture site and later atrophy of the immobilized limb result in a significant change in the limb circumference, leading to loosening of the immobilization, which may be the primary reason for these frequent dislocations [43]. Besides these limitations, what makes traditional plaster cast orthoses a golden standard is the wide availability of resources and the simple fact that it is a quicker and more intuitive solution, cheaper than a 3D-printed orthosis. On the other hand, 3D-printed orthoses offer increased patient comfort through individualized modeling and production. The advantages of this approach primarily include increased patient satisfaction with 3D-printed orthoses [35]. Additionally, its water-resistant and well-ventilated design facilitates better hygiene [44]. Proper fracture-site fixation is enabled not only by the personalized shape of the orthosis but also by its ability to be tightened [32] through the utilization of various bands, Velcro straps, or screws [45].

Those benefits come with a range of potential challenges associated with different 3D printing techniques, material options, and various modeling software and design solutions used for personalized orthoses (**Table 1**). Some of the major limitations of this innovative orthopedic approach are:

- It involves relatively expensive equipment (the price range of the equipment can vary from several thousand to several hundred thousand dollars);
- It often requires custom-made or expensive commercial surface scanners [45], to avoid patient exposure to radiological scans in order to acquire the surface 3D model of the fractured limb;
- There is a lack of highly skilled personnel who can adequately and quickly perform tasks such as surface 3D scanning, virtual modeling, 3D printing, and postprocessing of the 3D-printed objects.

Reference	3D printing technique	Material	3D printer /3D acquisition scanner	Used software	Study design	Reported time frame
Chen et al. [45]	Selective laser sintering	Polyamide 2,200	**3D printer** – EOS P395, (EOS GmbH Electro Optical Systems, Krailling, Germany) **CT** – Aquillion 64 (Toshiba, Japan) **MRI** – Achieva 1.5 or 3.0 T (Philips, Netherlands)	• Mimics10.01 (Materialise, Belgium); • Workbench 18.0 (ANSYS, USA); • SolidWorks 2015 (Dassault, France)	• 60 patients; • distal forearm fracture; • orthosis	3 to 5 days
Song et al. [47].	Fused deposition modeling	Polylactic acid	**3D printer** – Creality FDM 3D printer, model not specified (Shenzhen Creality 3D Technology Co. Ltd, China) **CT** – model not specified	• Mimics Research 19.0 (Materialise, Belgium); • Geomagic Studio (Raindrop, USA); • Rhino 6 (Robert McNeel, USA)	• 32 patients; • displaced intra-articular calcaneus fractures; • cast/ surgical guide	minimum 48 hours
Xiao et al. [48]	Fused deposition modeling	Polyester	**3D printer** – BY-3D-I instant 3D external fixation printer (Wuhan Biying Biological Technology Co. Ltd, China) **Surface 3D scanner** – EinScan pro 2x 3D scanner (Shining 3D, China)	• BY-3D-I instant printer slicing system (Wuhan Biying Biotechnology Co. Ltd, China)	• 40 patients; • Colles fracture; • orthosis	25 minutes
Guebeli et al. [49]	Digital light processing	Photosensitive resin (Immob A300 photopolymer resin)	**3D printer** – Atum 3D DLP Station (Gouda, Netherlands) **CT** – model not specified **Surface 3D scanner** – iPad 6th Generation (Apple Inc, USA); using an optical structure sensor (Mark I Structure Sensor; Occipital Inc, USA).	• Spentys SA/NV (Spentys SA, Brussels, Belgium)	• 39 patients; • distal radius fractures; • orthosis	3 to 5 days post-trauma
Hoogervorst et al. [50]	Multi Jet Fusion	HP PA12 Nylon	**3D printer** – HP Multi Jet Fusion Printer (Palo Alto, USA); model not specified **Radiology method** – Fluoroscopy **Surface 3D scanner** – 3D infrared Structure Sensor (Occipital Inc, USA), requires an iPad or other high-performance tablet to run;	• DPC (Standard Cyborg, USA)	• 8 cadavers; • distal radius fractures; • orthosis	not applicable
Tobler-Ammann et al. [51]	Selective laser sintering	Not specified	**3D printer** – type not specified **Surface 3D scanner** – HandySCAN 300 (Creaform, Canada)	Not specified	• 19 patients; • distal radius fractures; • orthosis	10.7 days on average

Table 1.
Contemporary studies focused on using personalized 3D-printed orthoses in individuals with bone fractures.

Further difficulties that impair the clinical use of 3D-printed orthoses lie in the total time required to obtain and place the 3D-printed orthosis [41]. While waiting for the entire process to be completed (**Figure 1**), the patient also requires immobilization, which is achieved with a traditional plaster orthosis. As shown in **Table 1**, in cases where an *in-house* bioengineering laboratory was used, an appointment for 3D-printed orthosis fitting is scheduled after 24 to 48 hours [38], and where a remote 3D printing laboratory was used, after 7 days [45]. The second approach requires additional patient appointments and even additional radiography to verify that there was no displacement of the fracture after removal of the plaster and application of a 3D-printed orthosis. Moreover, during clinical trials on 3D-printed orthoses for distal radius and forearm fractures, CT scanning of the contralateral hand [46] or even for both hands [45] was used. This is reasoned by the fact that an inadequate surface 3D scan may be obtained on a fractured limb due to swelling, and also because of the inability to hold the reduction position of the limb during surface 3D scan without external support (which would impair optical surface 3D scanning). Our approach to tackling this obstacle is to develop a software solution that can be implemented *in-house* to transform traditional radiographs into 3D models of the injured limb. Considering the methodological heterogeneity and design limitations of previous studies (**Table 1**), we advocate for the use of novel integrative approaches in further investigations on the clinical implementation of personalized 3D-printed orthoses in individuals with bone fractures.

5. Personalized 3D-printed orthoses in Serbia

During preparation for our ongoing clinical study (GovTech program), our team concluded that in a resource-limited healthcare system and under modest economic conditions in Serbia, we need to offer the additional value of 3D-printed personalized orthoses to motivate patients to undergo a more time-consuming and lengthy procedure to acquire them. Summarizing the previous chapter, we can state that the advantages of 3D-printed personalized orthoses for the forearm include increased patient satisfaction, enhanced comfort due to their water-resistant, well-ventilated, and lightweight construction, and some limited benefits from the adjustable fixation of the 3D-printed orthoses [32, 45]. However, apart from increased expenses, previous studies did not report a significant reduction in fracture healing time or total recovery time for the patients. With the intention of creating additional benefits for patients in the ongoing clinical study and generating potential benefits for the healthcare system, we decided to utilize the advantages enabled by the personalized orthosis design and introduce supplementary therapy in the form of therapeutic ultrasound and an electromagnetic field (EMF). Based on previous research, we developed a novel combination of adjunctive therapy, incorporating low-intensity pulsed ultrasound (LIPUS) and EMF under preplanned conditions tailored to each patient (**Figure 2**). We used a conventional ultrasound therapeutic frequency of 1.5 MHz [52] and an intensity of 30 mW/cm^2 [53], as well as an extremely low-frequency pulsed EMF with a peak amplitude intensity of 6.5 mT [54, 55]. Previous clinical studies and the principles of ultrasound propagation suggest that the therapeutic effects are most significant in cases of bone fractures near the skin surface [52]. In our ongoing clinical study, we virtually planned the orthosis to hold the small ultrasound

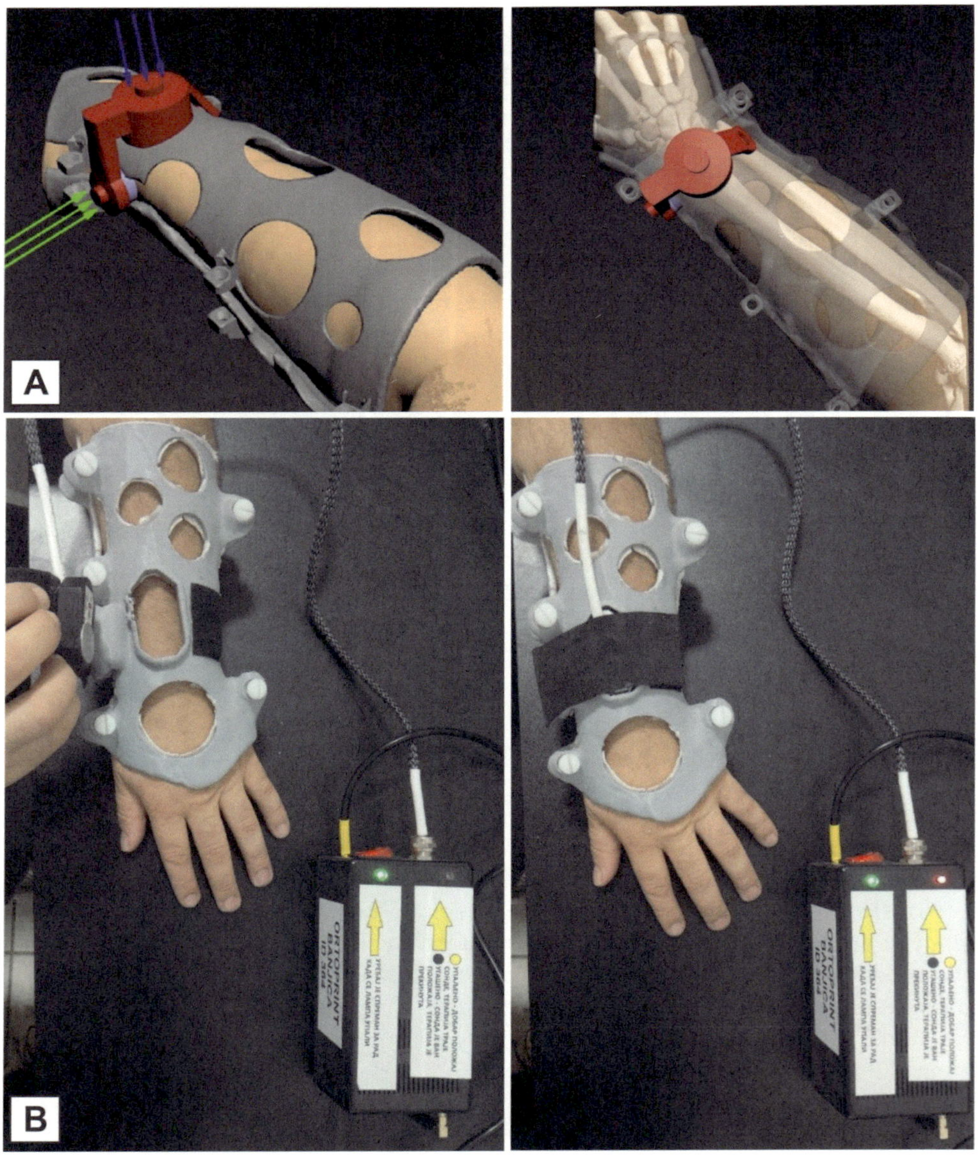

Figure 2.
Our solution for personalized 3D-printed orthoses with fitting supplementary therapy transducers of therapeutic ultrasound and electromagnetic field: virtual surgical planning (A) and therapy device (B).

transducer in place on the skin of the patient nearest to the fractured bone, and the EMF coil was integrated into the orthosis design in the position that enabled EMF to effectively reach the fracture site perpendicular to the direction of LIPUS propagation (**Figure 2A**). Having in mind that obligatory daily visits to the clinic would significantly reduce compliance of the patients included in the study, and considering the relatively low number of patients enrolled in previous clinical studies [55, 56], we designed and produced a portable device for LIPUS and EMF therapy with the possibility of remote therapy registration and monitoring

(**Figure 2B**). In this way, we have enabled patients to follow the study protocol from the convenience of their own homes, while we can remotely monitor their compliance via a dedicated server and application. By advancing the use of 3D-printed orthoses and adjunct therapies, including LIPUS and EMF, we aim to reduce fracture healing time [52] and conservatively treat a significant portion of non-union fractures [53, 54, 56], thereby alleviating some pressure on the Serbian healthcare system.

Another issue in the personalized 3D-printed orthosis production process, which became apparent after producing and implementing more than 20 orthoses during our clinical study, is the gap between the scanning procedure and the acquisition of the orthosis 3D model. As mentioned above, the majority of papers listed CT scanning as the source for 3D model acquisition; some also used, additionally or exclusively, different kinds of surface 3D scanners. The issue with 3D scanning is the additional radiation dose it imposes on the patient. The issue with optical surface scanning of the injured limb, specifically regarding distal radius fractures, is the inability of the patient to hold the fracture reduction position without external support, and it is also risky to try to hold the limb manually in the required position while acquiring the scan because of questionable repeatability and possible movements of the fractured bone fragments [47]. To overcome this issue, in the course of our clinical study, we implemented statistical shape models and an OpenGL-based software solution, a concept based on previous work of Ehlke et al. [57] for acquiring 3D models of forearm soft tissue profiles from DICOM data of 2D radiography, which is a standard procedure in distal forearm fracture diagnostics.

6. Conclusion

In summary, this chapter introduced the reader to the specific challenges of an innovative orthopedic approach involving the use of 3D printing in Serbia, with special emphasis on highlighting certain advantages and disadvantages of available 3D printing technologies in medicine. Without CAD/CAM, the full potential of personalized medicine in orthopedics would remain unrealized, hampered by inefficiencies and inaccuracies that these technologies adeptly overcome, paving the way for a future where every treatment is as unique as the patient it serves. Considering the limited clinical application of 3D printing in orthopedics, future interdisciplinary studies highlighting the cooperation between orthopedic surgeons, engineers, prosthetists, and physiatrists are warranted to reach its full clinical potential.

Acknowledgments

Authors received financial support from the Innovation Fund of the Republic of Serbia (Orthoprint group, GovTech program). Furthermore, Jelena Jadzic acknowledges the financial support from the Ministry of Science of the Republic of Serbia (support to the Center of Bone Biology as the center of excellence [Grant No. 451-03-1524/2023-04/18] and institutional funding to the Faculty of Medicine, University of Belgrade [Grant No. 451-03-137/2025-03/200110]).

Conflict of Interest

The authors declare that they have no conflicts of interest. The funding sources had no role in the writing or in the decision to publish the chapter.

Author details

Milutin Micic[1], Branislav Krivokapic[2] and Jelena Jadzic[1]*

1 Center of Bone Biology, Faculty of Medicine, University of Belgrade, Belgrade, Serbia

2 Institute of Orthopedics "Banjica", Faculty of Medicine, University of Belgrade, Belgrade, Serbia

*Address all correspondence to: jelena.jadzic@med.bg.ac.rs

References

[1] Prządka M, Pająk W, Kleinrok J, Pec J, Michno K, Karpiński R, et al. Advances in 3D printing applications for personalized orthopedic surgery: From anatomical modeling to patient-specific implants. Journal of Clinical Medicine 2025;**14**:3989

[2] Tack P, Victor J, Gemmel P, Annemans L. 3D-printing techniques in a medical setting: A systematic literature review. Biomedical Engineering Online. 2016;**15**(1):115

[3] Micic M, Djuric M. Acellular 3D printing in bone defect surgical reconstruction. Medical Youth. 2023;**74**(3):44–51

[4] Todd EA, Mirsky NA, Silva BLG, Shinde AR, Arakelians ARL, Nayak VV, et al. Functional scaffolds for bone tissue regeneration: A comprehensive review of materials, methods, and future directions. Journal of Functional Biomaterials 2024;**15**:280

[5] Sun J, Chen C, Zhang B, Yao C, Zhang Y. Advances in 3D-printed scaffold technologies for bone defect repair: Materials, biomechanics, and clinical prospects. Biomedical Engineering Online. 2025;**24**(1):51

[6] Jaiswal R, Wadetwar R. Technique of 3D printing for scaffolding in tissue engineering of bones: Opportunities and challenges. Materials Today Communications. 2025;**42**:111249

[7] Jadzic J, Djuric M. Structural basis of increased bone fragility in aged individuals: Multi-scale perspective. Medical Research. 2024;**57**(1): 67–74

[8] Albrektsson T, Johansson C. Osteoinduction, osteoconduction and osseointegration. European Spine Journal. 2001;**10**:S96–101

[9] García-Aznar JM, Nasello G, Hervas-Raluy S, Pérez MÁ, Gómez-Benito MJ. Multiscale modeling of bone tissue mechanobiology. Bone. 2021;**151**:116032

[10] Shen C, Witek L, Flores RL, Tovar N, Torroni A, Coelho PG, et al. Three-dimensional printing for craniofacial bone tissue engineering. Tissue Engineering Part A 2020;**26**:1303–1311

[11] Micic M, Antonijevic D, Milutinovic-Smiljanic S, Trisic D, Colovic B, Kosanovic D, et al. Developing a novel resorptive hydroxyapatite-based bone substitute for over-critical size defect reconstruction: Physicochemical and biological characterization and proof of concept in segmental rabbit's ulna reconstruction. Biomedizinische Technik (Berlin) 2020;**65**:491–505

[12] Andrés-Cano P, Calvo-Haro JA, Fillat-Gomà F, Andrés-Cano I, Perez-Mañanes R. Role of the orthopaedic surgeon in 3D printing: Current applications and legal issues for a personalized medicine. Rev Esp Cir Ortop Traumatol [Internet]. 2021;**65**(2):138–151. Available from: https://www.elsevier.es/es-revista-revista-espanola-cirugia-ortopedica-traumatologia-429-articulo-role-orthopaedic-surgeon-in-3d-S1988885621000018

[13] Ondrejova B, Stefanovic B, Rajtukova V, Zivcak J. Design and production of personalized cervical orthosis using CAD/CAM systems. Acta Tecnología. 2024;**10**(4):109–113

[14] Wong KC, Kumta SM, Leung KS, Ng KW, Ng EWK, Lee KS. Integration of CAD/CAM planning into computer assisted orthopaedic surgery. Computer Aided Surgery. 2010;**15**(4–6):65–74

[15] Hegele J, Seitz L, Claussen C, Baumert U, Sabbagh H, Wichelhaus A. Clinical effects with customized brackets and CAD/CAM technology: A prospective controlled study. Progress in Orthodontics. 2021;**22**(1):40

[16] Ejnisman L, Gobbato B, de França Camargo AF, Zancul E. Three-dimensional printing in orthopedics: From the basics to surgical applications. Current Reviews in Musculoskeletal Medicine. 2021;**14**:1–8

[17] Serrano C, Van Den Brink H, Pineau J, Prognon P, Martelli N. Benefits of 3D printing applications in jaw reconstruction: A systematic review and meta-analysis. Journal of Cranio-Maxillo -Facial Surgery. 2019;**4**(9):1387–1397

[18] Ballard DH, Mills P, Duszak R, Weisman JA, Rybicki FJ, Woodard PK. Medical 3D printing cost-savings in orthopedic and maxillofacial surgery: Cost analysis of operating room time saved with 3D printed anatomic models and surgical guides. Academic Radiology. 2020;**27**(8):1103–1113

[19] Wong KC. 3D-printed patient-specific applications in orthopedics. Orthopedic Research and Reviews. 2016;**8**:57–66

[20] Wu Y, Liu J, Kang L, Tian J, Zhang X, Hu J, et al. An overview of 3D printed metal implants in orthopedic applications: Present and future perspectives. Heliyon 2023;**9**:e17718

[21] Della Bona A, Cantelli V, Britto VT, Collares KF, Stansbury JW. 3D printing restorative materials using a stereolithographic technique: A systematic review. Dental Materials. 2021;**37**(2):336–350

[22] Meng M, Wang J, Huang H, Liu X, Zhang J, Li Z. 3D printing metal implants in orthopedic surgery: Methods, applications and future prospects. Journal of Orthopaedic Translation. 2023;**42**:94–112

[23] Micic M, Jadzic J, Milenkovic P, Antic S, Antonijevic D, Djuric MP. Testing of different scanning protocols used for precise 3D-printing of mandibular models. Journal of Craniofacial Surgery. 2023;**34**(7): e623–6. DOI: 10.1097/scs.0000000000009421

[24] Chen D, Zheng L, Wang C, Huang Y, Huang H, Apicella A, et al. Evaluation of surgical placement accuracy of customized CAD/CAM titanium mesh using screws-position-guided template: A retrospective comparative study. Clinical Implant Dentistry and Related Research 2023;**25**:519–531

[25] Jelovac D, Micic M, Hajdarevic S, Kuzmanovic C, Cukic B, Stefanovic B, et al. Immediate placement of extra-short implants in refined scapula tip microvascular free flaps: In house virtual planning and surgical technique – Proof of concept. Heliyon 2023;**9**:e18021

[26] Hsiao YC, De CC, Wu YH, Fang JJ. Anatomical-based customized cervical orthosis design in automation. Applied Sciences. 2024;**14**(16):7424

[27] Wu LN, Zhang ZF, Li RJ, Xin DQ, Wang JF. 3D printing for personalized solutions in cervical spondylosis. Orthopedic Research and Reviews. 2024;**16**:251–259

[28] Andres A, Roland M, Wickert K, Diebels S, Stöckl J, Herrmann S, et al. Advantages of digital twin technology in orthopedic trauma surgery – Exploring different clinical use cases. Scientific Reports. 2025;**15**(1):19987

[29] Salgado Manrique JS, Cifuentes-de la Portilla C. Exploring opportunities for advancements in lower limb socket fabrication and testing: A review. Biomechanics. 2025;**5**(3):64. Available from: https://www.mdpi.com/2673-7078/5/3/64

[30] Frizziero L, Pagliari C, Donnici G, Liverani A, Santi GM, Papaleo P, et al. Effectiveness assessment of CAD simulation in complex orthopedic surgery practices. Symmetry (Basel) 2021;**13**:850

[31] Stojkovic M, Trajanovic M, Vitkovic N. Personalized orthopedic surgery design challenge: Human bone redesign method. In: Putnik, Goran. Procedia CIRP. Póvoa de Varzim, Portgal: Elsevier B.V.; 2019. p. 701–706. DOI: 10.1016/j.procir.2019.04.170

[32] Popa DL, Buciu G, Calin DC, Popkonstantinović B, CAD PF. CAE and rapid prototyping methods applied in long bones orthopaedics. FME Transactions. 2019;**47**(2):279–286

[33] Micic M Influence of the Choice of Protocols on the Accuracy of Three-dimensional Medical Models, Surgical Guides and Bone Replacement [Internet] [PhD Thesis]. [Belgrade, Serbia]: University of Belgrade, Faculty of Medicine; 2023. Available from: https://phaidrabg.bg.ac.rs/detail/o:31360

[34] Eurostat. EU population structure and ageing [Internet]. https://ec.europa.eu/eurostat/statistics-explained/index.php?title=Population_structure_and_ageing#:~:text=update:%20February%202026.-,Highlights,aged%2065%20years%20and%20over. 2025. Available from: https://ec.europa.eu/eurostat/statistics-explained/index.php?title=Population_structure_and_ageing#:~:text=update:%20February%202026.-,Highlights,aged%2065%20years%20and%20over [Accessed: 2025-September-15]

[35] Institute for Public Health of Serbia. Health indicators in the Republic of Serbia - data presentation system [Internet]. https://www.batut.org.rs/download/zdravstveni_pokazatelji_rs_2020.html. 2021. Available from: https://www.batut.org.rs/download/zdravstveni_pokazatelji_rs_2020.html [Accessed: 2025-September-15]

[36] Gatt A, Formosa C, Chockalingam N. The application of generic CAD/CAM systems for the design and manufacture of foot orthoses. The Foot and Ankle Online Journal. 2016;**9**(3):6. Available from: https://faoj.org/2016/08/31/the-application-of-generic-cadcam-systems-for-the-design-and-manufacture-of-foot-orthoses/

[37] Mounsef PJ, Mulé P, Bernstein M, Hamdy R. The use of 3D printing as an educational tool in orthopaedics. JBJS Open Access. 2025;**10**(2):e25.00062

[38] Lazzeri S, Talanti E, Basciano S, Barbato R, Fontanelli F, Uccheddu F, et al. 3D-printed patient-specific casts for the distal radius in children: Outcome and pre-market survey. Materials 2022;**15**:2863

[39] Klopfer T, Hemmann P, Rupprecht V, Stuby F, Stöckle U, Meder A. Outcome analysis of distal radius fracture with orthosis versus cast immobilization after palmar plate osteosynthesis: A randomized

controlled study. Journal of Personalized Medicine. 2023;**13**(1):130

[40] Popescu D, Lăptoiu D, Căruțașu NL. Considerations on the design, printability and usability of customized 3D-printed upper limb orthoses. Applied Sciences. 2024;**14**(14):6157

[41] Oud T, Kerkum Y, De Groot P, Gijsbers H, Nollet F, Brehm MA. Production time and user satisfaction of 3-dimensional printed orthoses for chronic hand conditions compared with conventional orthoses: A prospective case series. Journal of Rehabilitation Medicine Clinical Communications. 2021;**4**:1000048

[42] Beumer A, McQueen MM. Fractures of the distal radius in low-demand elderly patients: Closed reduction of no value in 53 of 60 wrists. Acta Orthopaedica Scandinavica. 2003;**74**(1):98–100

[43] Janzing HMJ, Bessems SAM, Ligthart MAP, Van Lieshout EMM, Theeuwes HP, Barten DG, et al. Treatment of dorsally dislocated distal radius fractures with individualized 3D printed bracing: An exploratory study. 3D Printing in Medicine 2020;**6**:22

[44] Schwartz DA, Schofield KA. Utilization of 3D printed orthoses for musculoskeletal conditions of the upper extremity: A systematic review. Journal of Hand Therapy. 2023;**36**(1):166–178

[45] Chen Y, Lin H, Yu Q, Zhang X, Wang D, Shi L, et al. Application of 3D-printed orthopedic cast for the treatment of forearm fractures: Finite element analysis and comparative clinical assessment. BioMed Research International. 2020;**2020**:9569530

[46] Van Lieshout EMM, Verhofstad MHJ, Beens LM, Van Bekkum JJJ, Willemsen F, Janzing HMJ, et al. Personalized 3D-printed forearm braces as an alternative for a traditional plaster cast or splint; A systematic review. Injury 2022;**53**:S47–52

[47] Song Q, Li T, Xia H, Li Y, Feng C, Lin Y, et al. Three-dimensional printed cast assisted screw fixation of calcaneal fractures: A prospective study. BMC Musculoskeletal Disorders 2023;**24**:802

[48] Xiao YP, Xu HJ, Liao W, Li ZH. Clinical application of instant 3D printed cast versus polymer orthosis in the treatment of colles fracture: A randomized controlled trial. BMC Musculoskeletal Disorders. 2024;**25**(1):104

[49] Guebeli A, Thieringer F, Honigmann P, Keller M. In-house 3D-printed custom splints for non-operative treatment of distal radial fractures: A randomized controlled trial. Journal of Hand Surgery. 2024;**49**(3):350–358. DOI: 10.1177/17531934231187554

[50] Hoogervorst P, Knox R, Tanaka K, Working ZM, El Naga AN, Herfat S, et al. A biomechanical comparison of fiberglass casts and 3-dimensional–printed, open-latticed, ventilated casts. Hand 2020;**15**:842–849

[51] Tobler-Ammann B, Schuind F, Voillat L, Vögelin E. Acceptability and safety of 3D printed wrist-based orthoses compared to fiberglass casts for the treatment of non-surgical distal radius- and scaphoid fractures: A randomized feasibility trial. Journal of Hand Therapy. 2025;**38**(1):143–151. DOI: 10.1016/j.jht.2024.11.004

[52] Mundi R, Petis S, Kaloty R, Shetty V, Bhandari M. Low-intensity pulsed ultrasound: Fracture healing. Indian Journal of Orthopaedics. 2009;**43** (2):132–140. Available from: https://pmc.ncbi.nlm.nih.gov/articles/PMC2762261/

[53] Busse JW, Bhandari M, Kulkarni AV, Tunks E. The effect of low-intensity pulsed ultrasound therapy on time to fracture healing: A meta-analysis. CMAJ. 2002;**166**(4): 437–441. Available from: https://www.cmaj.ca/content/166/4/437.long

[54] Ehnert S, Schröter S, Aspera-Werz RH, Eisler W, Falldorf K, Ronniger M, et al. Translational insights into extremely low frequency pulsed electromagnetic fields (ELF-PEMFs) for bone regeneration after trauma and orthopedic surgery. Journal of Clinical Medicine 2019;**8**:2028

[55] Lazović M, Kocić M, Dimitrijević L, Stanković I, Spalević M, Affiliations TC, et al. Pulsed electromagnetic field during cast immobilization in postmenopausal women with Colles' fracture. Srp Arh Celok Lek 2012;**140**:619–624

[56] Martinez-Rondanelli A, Martinez JP, Moncada ME, Manzi E, Pinedo CR, Cadavid H. Electromagnetic stimulation as coadjuvant in the healing of diaphyseal femoral fractures: A randomized controlled trial. Colomb Med (Cali). 2014;**45**(2):67–71

[57] Ehlke M, Ramm H, Lamecker H, Hege HC, Zachow S. Fast generation of virtual X-ray images for reconstruction of 3D anatomy. IEEE Transactions on Visualization and Computer Graphics. 2013;**19**(12):2673–2682

Section 2

Fracture Management in Special Populations and Anatomical Regions

Chapter 3

Acetabular Fractures in the Elderly

Fernando Antunez-Muiños, Alberto Jorge-Mora, Tamara de la Rasilla-Sainz, Belen Ines Vieira-Lopez, Diego Novillo-Casal, Jorge González-García, Felipe Ignacio Vergara-Gutiérrez and Iván Castro-Arias

Abstract

Acetabular fractures in elderly patients are an increasingly frequent consequence of population aging. Although commonly caused by low-energy falls, they are associated with high morbidity and mortality, approaching 20% at one year, largely due to patient frailty and comorbidities. Fracture patterns typically involve the anterior column with posterior hemitransverse and acetabular dome injury, with medial protrusion and superomedial impaction (gull sign), features that predict poor outcomes with conventional reconstruction. Management requires a multidisciplinary orthogeriatric approach focused on early stabilization, pain control, and individualized treatment selection. Conservative management is reserved for stable or minimally displaced fractures and high-risk surgical candidates, avoiding perioperative complications but carrying the risk of functional limitation and late conversion to total hip arthroplasty (THA). Open reduction and internal fixation (ORIF) offer good results when anatomic reduction is achieved, though with high complication and reoperation rates. In recent years, combined fixation with acute arthroplasty (fix and replace) has gained support for complex osteoporotic fractures, reducing reoperations and providing comparable function to ORIF. Overall, outcomes depend more on achieving pain-free hip stability than on the specific technique. Treatment should be individualized, balancing surgical risk, fracture anatomy, and patient condition to optimize mobility and quality of life.

Keywords: acetabular fracture, ORIF, total hip replacement, elderly, surgical treatment

1. Introduction, epidemiology, and mechanism of injury

Acetabular fractures in the elderly represent a minority but growing percentage of all acetabular fractures, with an increasing proportion in recent years, rising from less than 10% of the total to almost a quarter of all such fractures [1]. One of the largest series from Matta et al. demonstrates an increase in the mean age from 32 in the 1980s to 49 years old at the end of the first decade of the twenty-first century [1]. Epidemiological studies indicate that they constitute only ~1.5–3% of all skeletal injuries, but their incidence has increased ~2.4 times over the past three decades due to population aging [1, 2]. The reported mean age is usually around 70–80 years, with a high prevalence of comorbidities (over 80% present with significant medical conditions). The injury mechanism in older adults is typically low-energy (e.g., falls from standing height in ~80% of cases) rather than the high-energy trauma typical in younger patients. However, these fractures in the elderly are not trivial: they are associated with elevated short and medium-term mortality [3]. Various series report a one-year mortality between 14% and 25%, reaching even higher figures in patients managed non-surgically (especially those who are very frail and receive only traction) [2]. For example, in a trauma center, 33% of patients over 65 years old with acetabular fractures died within the first year, and the majority (84%) of those deaths occurred in patients managed non-surgically. In contrast, selected patients who underwent surgery had a lower mortality rate (around 12–15% at one year) in some cohorts, though this benefit may reflect a selection bias (healthier patients) [4]. In general, the patient's frailty and comorbidities play a central role in prognosis, and there is an emphasis on the need for comprehensive management (including orthogeriatric co-management) to optimize survival and functional recovery in elderly patients with acetabular fractures [2].

In patients over 65 years of age, most acetabular fractures result from low-energy mechanisms, typically falls from standing height, with the lower limb in extension or slight rotation. In such circumstances, the load transmitted through the femoral head impacts the roof or anterior wall of the acetabulum. This phenomenon reflects a combination of osteoporotic bone, reduced cushioning muscle mass, and a diminished ability to correct body position during a fall. For example, a recent German study reported that these low-energy traumas predominate in this age group and lead to fractures most frequently involving the anterior acetabular structures (anterior column, anterior wall, medial surface), as opposed to the high-energy patterns typically observed in younger adults. This pattern contrasts with that of young adults, in whom high-energy accidents (such as motor vehicle collisions or falls from height) predominate and commonly produce posterior wall or column fractures. The importance of recognizing this mechanism lies in several clinical implications: first, that low-energy trauma may be underestimated, leading to delayed diagnosis; second, that the presence of osteoporosis and acetabular dome impaction is associated with poorer fixation prognosis; and third, that therapeutic strategies should be adapted accordingly – for instance, considering more functional treatment options or early arthroplasty rather than directly applying protocols designed for younger adults [5, 6].

2. Classification and patterns

The classic classification by Letournel and Judet remains the reference for describing these fractures. It distinguishes five elementary patterns (e.g., posterior wall, anterior column, etc.) and five associated patterns (such as both columns, transverse-posterior, T-shaped, etc.). However, in patients over 65 years of age, a particular distribution of patterns and certain characteristic radiological features are observed:

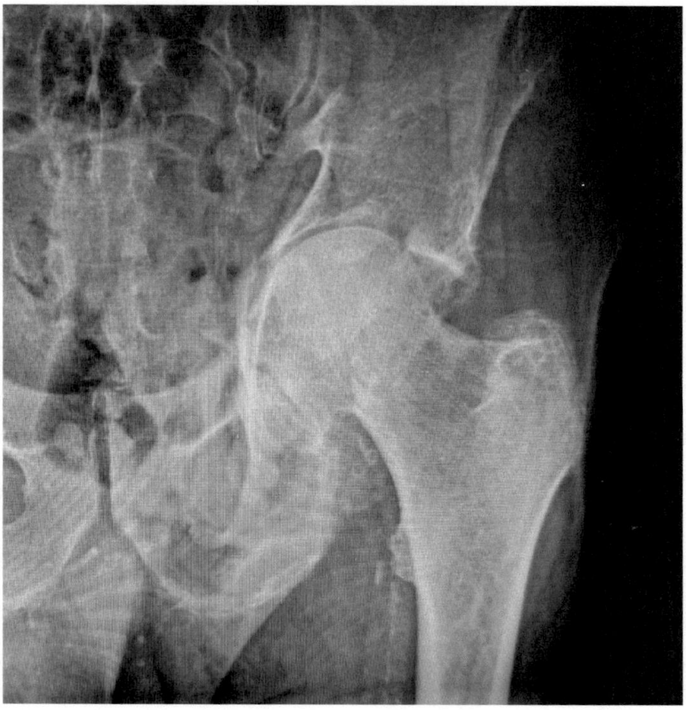

Figure 1.
Acetabular fracture (anterior and posterior hemitransverse).

- Most frequent patterns: Approximately two-thirds of acetabular fractures in elderly patients affect both columns (associated) or the anterior column with posterior hemitransverse. These patterns involve the acetabular roof and the quadrilateral surface, often with medial protrusion of the femoral head (**Figure 1**) [4].

- Fractures with impaction: Osteoporosis and bone fragility predispose individuals to impaction of the acetabular dome (roof), visible on Xrays/CT scans as the "gull sign" described by Anglen. This superomedial impaction is an adverse prognostic factor; initial studies showed that when present and not adequately reduced, internal fixation fails in nearly 100% of cases (early loss of reduction and arthritis). Therefore, the presence of comminution and dome impaction is associated with a high risk of failure of traditional reconstructive treatment and the subsequent need for arthroplasty [7, 8].

- Articular comorbidity: It is not uncommon for elderly patients to have pre-existing osteoarthritis or concomitant injuries (e.g., femoral head fracture) at the time of acetabular trauma, which influence the definitive treatment strategy [2, 4, 8].

In summary, elderly patients typically present with complex acetabular fractures (involving both columns) with osteoporotic bone fragments, and a tendency toward medial protrusion and marginal impaction. These factors necessitate individualized therapeutic strategies, as they complicate anatomic reduction and compromise the stability of traditional fixation methods [1, 2].

3. Initial management

The initial management of an acetabular fracture in patients over 65 years of age does not essentially differ from that of younger patients regarding the first measures, but it requires special consideration of the patient's overall condition:

- Attention to polytrauma: The patient should first be stabilized according to trauma protocols (ABCDE). Although many fractures in the elderly result from low-energy mechanisms, the possibility of other concomitant injuries should not be underestimated [9].

- Urgent reduction of dislocation: If the acetabular fracture is associated with a hip dislocation (e.g., in posterior wall fractures), urgent closed reduction should be performed to protect the viability of the articular cartilage [10].

- Immobilization and traction: In the acute phase, especially if surgical intervention is delayed, skeletal traction – trans-tibial or femoral – can be applied to relieve pain, maintain limb length, and prevent proximal migration of the femur. Temporary traction (generally 10–15 kg) helps prevent further protrusion of the femoral head in medial fractures [11, 12].

- Prophylaxis and medical support: Given the advanced age, it is crucial to initiate prophylaxis for deep vein thrombosis, provide effective analgesia, and ensure pulmonary care (to avoid complications due to immobility). Assessment by a geriatric team can optimize comorbidities (cardiac, metabolic) before possible surgery. A multidisciplinary orthogeriatric approach has been shown to reduce complications in hip fractures and is, by analogy, applicable to pelvis/acetabular injuries [13, 14].

- Early therapeutic decision-making: As soon as the patient's condition allows, the treating team (orthopedic surgeons together with geriatricians/anesthesiologists) must determine whether the patient will tolerate surgery or if conservative management will be chosen. Factors such as previous autonomy, cognitive status, comorbidities (cardiopulmonary insufficiency, etc.), and the fracture pattern (hip stability, articular displacement) influence this decision [8].

In summary, initial treatment combines general stabilization, pain relief, and fracture immobilization (usually with traction) while planning the most appropriate definitive strategy for each patient.

4. Definitive treatment

Definitive management of acetabular fractures in patients over 65 years of age can be grouped into conservative (non-surgical) and surgical approaches.

Within surgical management, there are several strategies: traditional osteosynthesis (open reduction and internal fixation), acute total hip arthroplasty (THA; either isolated or combined with fragment fixation, known as "fix and replace"), or intermediate approaches such as minimal percutaneous fixation. There is no absolute consensus on a single algorithm; the decision must be individualized, considering the fracture pattern and patient characteristics [1, 4, 8, 15–17]. A review of the options and their outcomes are discussed below.

5. Conservative treatment

Nonoperative management consists of observation, relative rest, and rehabilitation without open reduction. It is reserved for well-defined situations:

- Indications: Patients at very high surgical risk (advanced age, multiple severe comorbidities) or those with minimally displaced and stable fractures where the hip is expected to maintain reasonable congruence. In the literature, selection criteria include age >75 years, two or more major comorbidities, or non-displaced or impacted fractures in which the femoral head is "locked" in a stable position. A relatively frequent pattern in these conservatively managed patients is an isolated anterior column fracture (reported as 25% of nonoperatively managed cases) [1, 18].

- Protocol: This usually involves non-weight bearing for ~6–8 weeks (or protected partial weight bearing with a walker), analgesia, and physiotherapy for range of motion as pain allows. Radiographic monitoring is performed to ensure secondary displacement does not occur, with a control always indicated after sitting up with good pain control [15].

- Outcomes: Functional results are variable. In carefully selected patients (low displacement fractures and low functional demand), surprisingly acceptable outcomes have been reported – for example, a systematic review found that the nonoperatively managed group had an average Harris Hip Score (HHS) of ~93 at follow-up, the highest among the modalities analyzed. This reflects that many of these patients had relatively benign fractures or achieved "secondary congruence" of the hip. However, in more complex fractures, conservative treatment carries a risk of malunion and painful posttraumatic osteoarthritis. About 8% of patients initially managed nonoperatively required later conversion to THA due to pain and incongruity. Mortality in this group is high – about 18% at one year, and even up to 30–40% in some series of very frail patients who never recover from prolonged immobilization [4, 19, 20].

- Advantages and disadvantages: Its main advantage is avoiding surgical risks (anesthesia, bleeding, infection). In fact, nonoperative management showed the lowest rate of non-fatal complications in a recent meta-analysis. Nevertheless, this lower morbidity is countered by greater dependency: many patients do not regain independent ambulation after conservative treatment and require institutionalization or assistive devices. Furthermore, if the fracture consolidates incongruently, chronic pain and functional limitation may be significant [3, 4, 18, 20].

In conclusion, conservative management may be considered in selected elderly patients (minimally displaced fractures and/or inoperable patients) and can achieve acceptable results in those cases. However, it carries the risk of secondary osteoarthritis, and its indication should be evaluated on a case-by-case basis, weighing life expectancy and the patient's functional level.

6. Open reduction and internal fixation

Osteosynthesis via ORIF has been, for decades, the standard treatment for acetabular fractures, seeking to restore joint anatomy. In older patients, ORIF remains an important option, although technically more challenging and with less predictable results than in younger individuals:

- Patient and pattern selection: ORIF is considered when it is believed possible to achieve an anatomic or near-anatomic reduction of the articular surface, and the patient can tolerate surgery. This usually applies to more active and healthier elderly patients (65–75 years old, with reasonable life expectancy) and fractures that, though complex, are reconstructible (e.g., wall/column fractures with moderate comminution). In studies, around 35–40% of patients over 65 with acetabular fractures are treated with ORIF. There is also evidence supporting an adverse relationship between functional outcomes and body mass index [4, 21].

- Surgical technique: The concept does not differ from ORIF in younger patients; it requires adequate surgical exposure (using classic approaches such as anterior ilioinguinal or posterior Kocher–Langenbeck, and even combined or modified approaches if necessary). In geriatric series, about 69% of surgeries were performed via an anterior approach (for patterns involving the anterior column/ quadrilateral surface through posterior hemitransverse) and about 29% via a posterior approach (e.g., posterior wall fractures). Fixation usually includes plates and screws adapted for osteoporotic bone (e.g., use of infrapectineal plates for buttressing the medial quadrilateral surface, long iliac screws, etc.). Grafting of impaction areas with bone graft (generally from the femoral head or allograft) is recommended after elevating the impacted fragment of the acetabular dome to support the reduction [1, 4].

- Surgical approaches: The surgical approaches for acetabular fractures are selected based on the fracture pattern, fragment location, and the need for anatomical exposure. The most commonly used routes are the posterior (Kocher-Langenbeck), anterior (ilioinguinal), and extensile (extended iliofemoral) approaches. For instance, the Kocher-Langenbeck approach is considered the "workhorse" for posterior wall or column fractures because it provides excellent visualization of the posterior pillar and has been associated with low complication rates when appropriately indicated. The ilioinguinal approach is preferred for anterior column or wall fractures, as it allows access to the inner anterior pelvic surface and the acetabular face from the frontal aspect. The extensile iliofemoral approach provides comprehensive exposure of both columns and the acetabular roof, making it suitable for complex fractures (e.g., both-column or T-shaped patterns), but it carries greater morbidity (increased bleeding, risk of heterotopic ossification) and requires substantial surgical experience. In terms of clinical outcomes, the critical factor is not the chosen approach itself but the quality of the articular reduction achieved; nevertheless, selecting the appropriate approach facilitates this reduction, minimizes unnecessary operative time, and may reduce access-related complications. In recent years, there has been a progressive shift from traditional approaches for anterior column and posterior hemitransverse fractures toward intrapelvic and pararectus approaches. These anterior techniques offer the advantage of less muscle detachment while allowing, from their position, improved neutralization of the forces that tend to medialize the femoral head, facilitating the reduction of the fracture [22–30].

- Achievement of anatomic reduction: This is critical as it strongly influences prognosis. A recent study highlights that, in elderly operated patients, those in whom residual reduction ≤3 mm was achieved had markedly better results: lower rates of posttraumatic osteoarthritis (18% vs 77%), higher average Harris Hip Scores (82 vs 69 points), and were four times more likely to have a "good" clinical outcome compared to those with >3 mm incongruity. In other words, even in elderly patients, good articular reduction is associated with satisfactory results, whereas poor reductions carry clinical failure and may anticipate the need for a total hip replacement [8].

- Outcomes and complications: ORIF in older adults preserves the native joint and, if reduction is successful, can provide several years of good function. In general, patients operated on with ORIF reach mean Harris Hip Scores of ~80–85 in the mid-term, and many regain partial or complete weight-bearing ambulation. However, complication rates are not low; according to a systematic review, ORIF in the elderly displayed the highest rate of non-fatal complications compared to other modalities. These complications include wound infection, neurovascular injury, thrombosis, heterotopic ossification, fixation failure (loss of reduction), and the need for reoperation. A recent multicenter study reported that, at >5 years, approximately 20% of patients treated with ORIF required revision surgery (usually conversion to prosthesis) due to fixation failure or painful osteoarthritis. The presence of dome impaction (gull sign) is particularly ominous: Anglen et al. observed early failure (loss of reduction) in 7 of 10 elderly patients with superior impaction, and this characteristic was 100% predictive of isolated ORIF failure (**Figure 2**). Even with modern techniques (modified Stoppa intrapelvic approach), conversion rates to prosthesis remain ~33% when severe impaction exists [1, 7, 8, 15].

- Mortality and recovery: Surgery inherently carries perioperative risks (bleeding, anesthesia, nerve injury). Nevertheless, when surgical stabilization is achieved, earlier patient mobility is promoted, which can mitigate complications from immobility. Some studies suggest that operated patients survive longer than those managed conservatively in the short term, but recent meta-analyses do not find significant differences in mortality when adjusted for baseline condition. Most older patients operated on with ORIF do not regain their previous functional level: they often require permanent walkers or canes, and only a percentage return home unaided; many transition to prolonged rehabilitation or care facilities [1, 3, 15, 16].

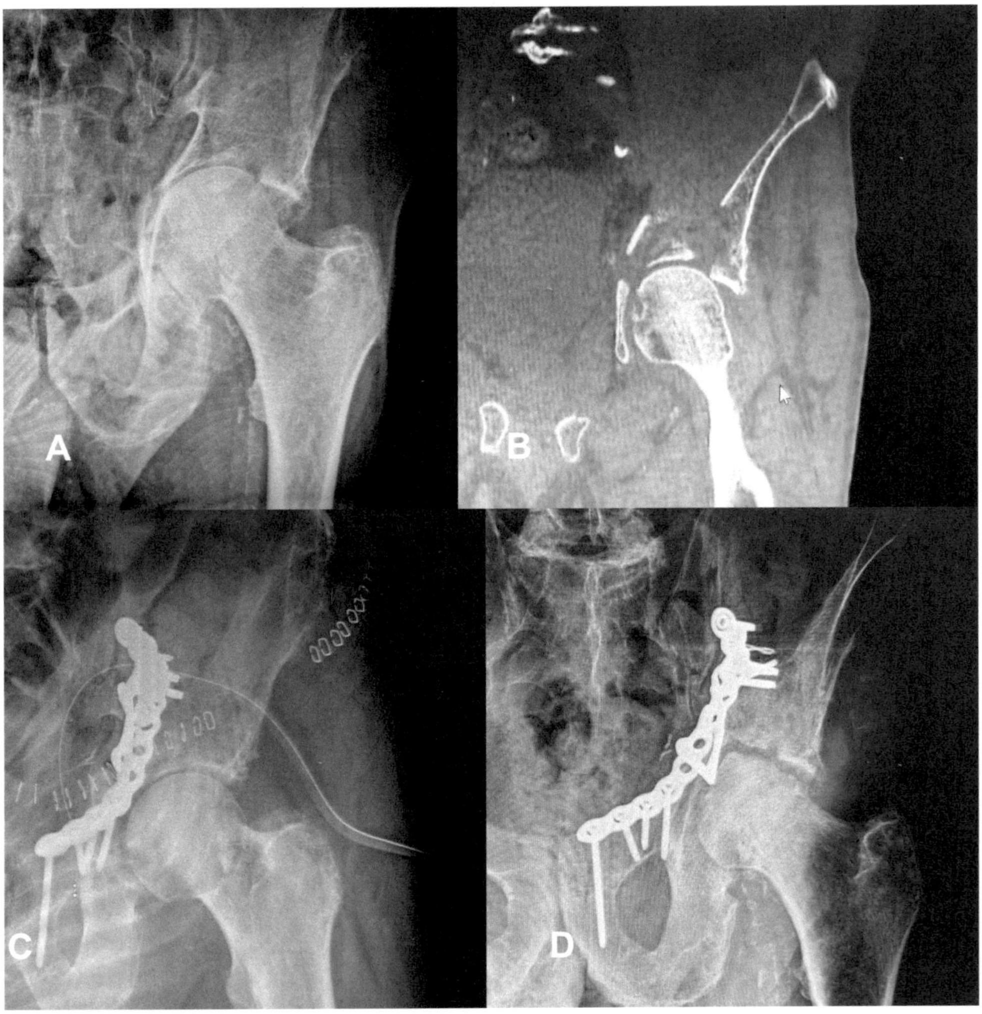

Figure 2.
(a): Fracture. (b): CT image of dome impaction and "gull sign." (c): Postoperative fixation. (d): Early failure after 5 months.

In summary, ORIF remains the mainstay in displaced fractures if the patient can tolerate it, with the premise of seeking the best possible reduction. It offers good functional results in elderly patients who achieve anatomic reduction but presents a significant complication rate, and about one in five may subsequently require rescue hip arthroplasty due to posttraumatic osteoarthritis or fixation failure.

7. Early total hip: "fix and replace"

Given the high failure rate of ORIF in osteoporotic bone (especially in the presence of chondral damage or impaction), combined surgical management has gained traction in recent years: performing acute THA together with fixation of the major acetabular fragments. This approach is sometimes called the "combined hip procedure" (CHP) or colloquially "fix and replace" [31].

- Indication: It is considered in elderly patients with complex acetabular fractures where the likelihood of achieving or maintaining an anatomic reduction is low and/or there is significant damage to the femoral head or cartilage. Typical examples include fractures with severe comminution of the acetabular dome (significant impaction, "gull sign"), fractures associated with femoral head necrosis or fracture, and very elderly patients (>75–80 years) in whom even a successful reduction may be frustrated by rapid arthritis. It is also considered in cases with pre-existing hip osteoarthritis. In these situations, performing primary THA may provide a definitive solution, avoiding a second future surgery [31].

- Technique: The principle is to stabilize the acetabular fracture sufficiently to implant a stable prosthetic acetabulum (**Figure 3**). This usually requires partial internal fixation: for example, reducing and fixing the posterior column if displaced, or placing an intrapelvic plate to contain the quadrilateral surface, etc., followed by implantation of a primary or revision acetabular cup. In highly comminuted fractures, reconstruction rings (cup-cage) or structural grafts may be used, but the trend is to use modern porous-coated cups. Key: To mitigate the high risk of prosthetic dislocation in this context, most surgeons opt for dual mobility cups in the acute arthroplasty, as they have been shown to reduce dislocation incidence in high-risk patients. The procedure is ideally performed through a single approach if possible: for example, many patterns can be treated completely through a posterior approach (Kocher-Langenbeck), first performing ORIF of the column/posterior wall and then implanting the prosthesis via

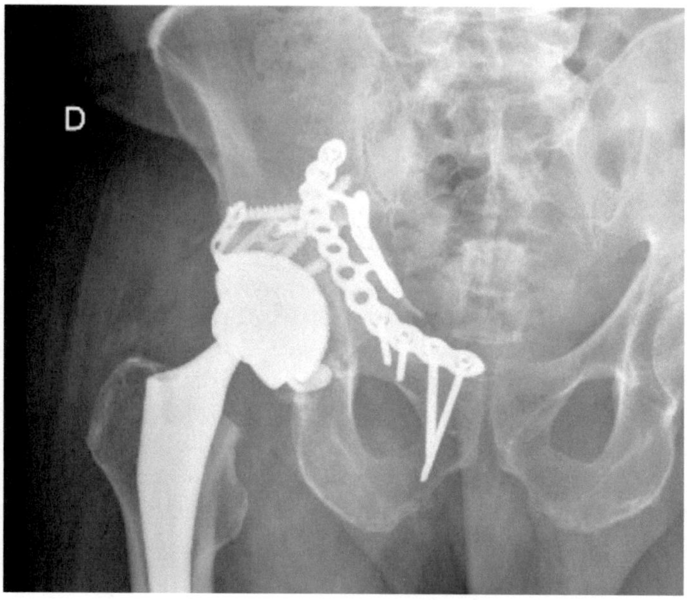

Figure 3.
Postoperative Xray of early fixation and replacement.

the same approach. This reduces operative time and complications compared to combining anterior and posterior approaches in the same session [16, 32].

- Outcomes: Recent evidence suggests that this combined strategy may offer equivalent or superior results to isolated ORIF in the elderly in terms of reoperations and satisfaction:

  - Several comparative (usually retrospective) studies show lower rates of subsequent surgical revisions when acute THA is performed versus ORIF alone. In a European study with ≥5 years of follow-up, the ORIF + THA group required revision in only ~7.7% of cases compared to 20% in ORIF alone. Another multicenter study observed no conversions to prosthesis in the combined procedure group versus ~10% early conversions in the pure ORIF group. This supports the idea that "fix and replace" avoids reoperations due to fixation failure [16, 33].

  - Functionally, outcomes and patient-reported outcome measures (PROMs) between ORIF and acute THA tend to be similar in the short to mid-term. Studies have found comparable Harris Hip Scores, SF-12 (quality of life), and Merle d'Aubigné scores between patients undergoing traditional ORIF versus combined procedures. For example, Smakaj et al. reported no significant differences in HHS or physical/mental SF-12 components at 2 and 5 years between groups. Lannes et al. also found mean HHS around 80 in both groups (no significant difference). Some improvements have been observed favoring the acute THA group: less chronic pelvic pain (lower pelvic discomfort index at 5 years) and better Oxford Hip Scores (average 40 vs. 33 points) compared to those who had delayed THA after failed ORIF. These data suggest that primary arthroplasty provides the patient with a definitively painless and stable joint from the outset, avoiding the stiffness/deterioration period experienced by those who fail and require late prosthesis implantation [16, 31, 33].

  - In terms of safety, surprisingly, the combined strategy does not substantially increase immediate risk compared to ORIF alone. Operative time and initial hospital stay were similar in one study, though there was a trend toward longer surgery with acute THA. Intraoperative blood loss tends to be higher in combined surgeries due to the dual procedure. Regarding complications, several analyses indicate that acute arthroplasty does not increase mortality (similar to ORIF) and may even have fewer non-fatal complications than ORIF. In one review, patients with ORIF + THA presented lower odds of complications compared to ORIF alone (OR 0.53); this may be because it avoids the "failure of reduction" complication inherent to ORIF. Of course, there are specific risks: prosthetic dislocation remains a major concern. Even with dual mobility cups, dislocation rates of ~8% have been reported in these combined patients. Deep infection risk may also increase slightly, given the greater magnitude of surgery (osteosynthesis plus prosthetic implantation in a traumatic field) [16, 20, 31, 33].

  - Special considerations: It is important to highlight the learning curve and planning required for this combined approach. It requires the availability of both a trauma surgeon and a joint replacement surgeon (or a team experienced in both) and suitable implants (pelvic plates, special cups, etc.). The concept, defended by some authors, is that in the presence of poor prognostic factors (e.g., fractured/impacted acetabular roof), it is preferable to "definitively solve" the hip in a single surgical stage. This avoids subjecting fragile patients to two major surgeries (an ORIF now and a rescue THA months later). In summary, evidence is consolidating in support of acute THA with fixation in selected older patients, achieving clinical results comparable to or better than ORIF and reducing reoperations in the medium term [32].

8. Late conversion to THA

The conversion rate varies depending on the initial management and present risk factors. In conservatively managed fractures, the need for late THA was about 8% in published series. After ORIF, literature reports a wider range: globally, about 10–30% of patients over 60 years end up with a prosthesis within the first 5–10 years post-fracture, being more likely in the presence of dome impaction (e.g., Anglen reported 100% conversion with massive impaction, and Laflamme about 33% with improved intrapelvic technique). Even minimally invasive percutaneous fixation (closed reduction and percutaneous pinning – CRPP) – sometimes used in very frail elderly – carries a high rate of subsequent arthroplasty; a meta-analysis indicated that patients with CRPP had a higher likelihood of requiring THA than non-operated patients (OR 2.15 vs. conservative) and more than conventional ORIF [1, 3, 7, 20, 32, 33].

Delayed THA performed long after the fracture represents a greater surgical challenge than a standard primary THA. There are scars and altered planes from previous surgery (if ORIF was done, partial or total implant removal is often necessary, and in some situations performed through different approaches). Acetabular deformity and bone loss may exist (from fracture or bone collapse). These revision surgeries pose higher risks of bleeding, infection, nerve damage, and dislocation (**Figure 4**). Therefore, the use of special cups (dual mobility or anti-protrusion rings) is usually recommended to improve stability in these late conversions [34–36].

Functionally, evidence suggests that patients who undergo late THA tend to have worse statuses than those who received the prosthesis initially. For example, Nicol et al. found that patients who had failed ORIF followed by THA had worse average Oxford Hip Scores (~33 points) compared with similar patients who had acute THA (~40 points). This reflects that those patients endured a period of limitation and pain before conversion, possibly suffering from sarcopenia or functional loss in the interim. However, once conversion is performed, many patients achieve significant pain relief and some functional improvement, although complication rates are not negligible (deep infections, dislocations, and re-revisions are more frequent than in primary arthroplasties) [3, 21, 33–36].

In conclusion, conversion to THA is a common salvage strategy in elderly patients with acetabular fractures. Ideally, it is anticipated who will require it to offer early rather than late surgery. When needed, it must be performed with appropriate reconstructive techniques (possibly using dual-mobility cups, grafts/supports, or revision cups) to achieve the best possible function.

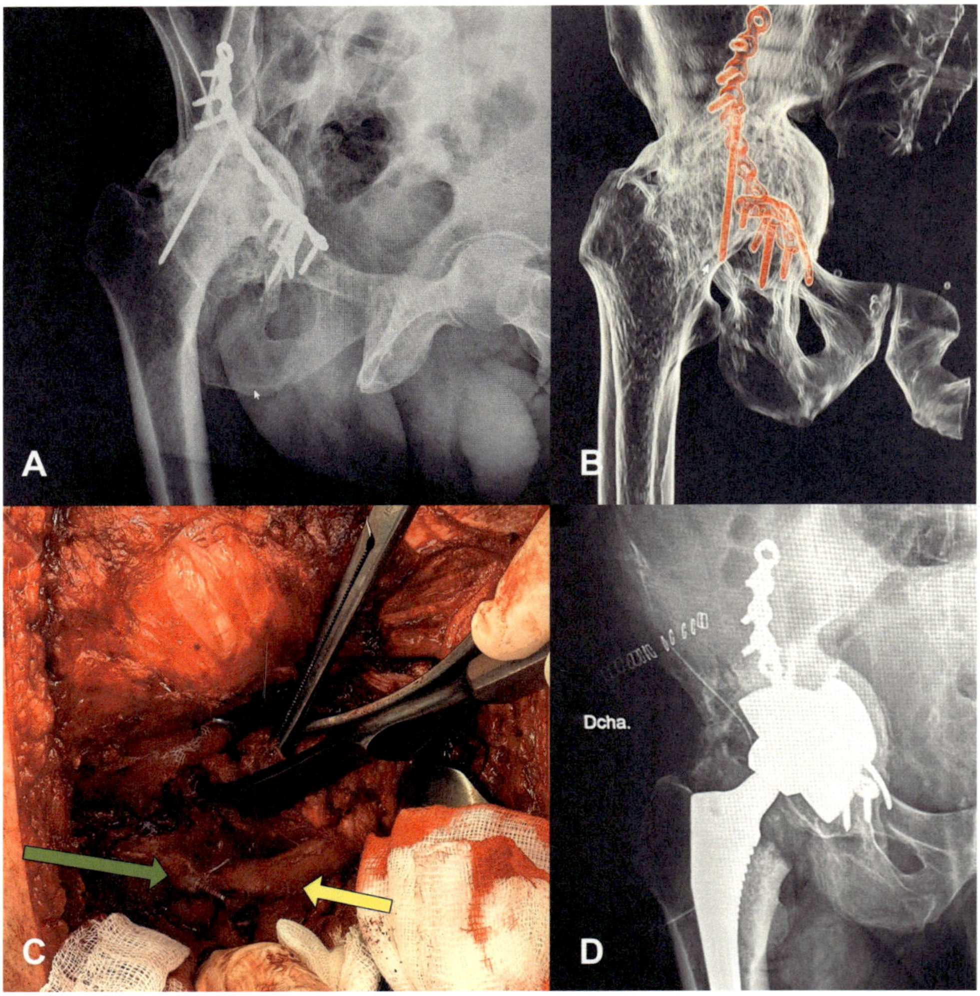

Figure 4.
a: Preoperative Xray prior late replacement. b: CT reconstruction of the hip. c: Intraoperative image of the sciatic nerve damaged by screw. d: Postoperative Xray.

9. Outcomes, rehabilitation, and PROMs

The evaluation of outcomes in this context includes objective clinical measures (consolidation, range of motion, need for walking aids) and functional scales, many of which are patient-reported outcome measures (PROMs). The main findings over the past 20 years indicate:

- Quality of life and overall function: Overall, many elderly patients with acetabular fractures do not fully regain their previous mobility level. At approximately 2–3 years post-injury, mean Harris Hip Scores (HHS) are around 80–85 points (out of 100) in those treated surgically, indicating good to moderate function but with some limitations. Interestingly, aggregated analyses found that the non-operated group had a higher mean HHS (~93), likely due to selection bias, as only patients with very minimally symptomatic fractures remained untreated. Prospective studies find that the key factor is the quality of the articular reduction rather than the treatment method itself: patients with anatomic reduction have significantly higher HHS than those with poor reduction, regardless of ORIF or prosthesis [3, 8, 21].

- Specific PROMs: Various outcome questionnaires have been employed, including the Oxford Hip Score (OHS), SF-12 Health Survey, WOMAC, and EuroQoL-5D. In general, no drastic long-term differences are observed between treatment modalities in comparable patients. For example, the OHS was significantly better (40 vs. 34, on a 0–48 scale where higher is better) in elderly patients receiving acute arthroplasty versus delayed ORIF. A study also found that the Pelvic Discomfort Index (PDI) at 5 years was lower (better) in patients with acute prostheses compared to those with ORIF. Conversely, other measures, such as SF-12 (physical and mental components), showed no significant difference between ORIF and combined treatment groups, suggesting that self-reported quality of life may be similar as long as the final outcome (with or without prosthesis) provides a pain-free hip [31, 33].

- Once the fracture has been stabilized – and particularly following surgical intervention – older patients require an adapted rehabilitation protocol that prioritizes early mobilization, progressive weight-bearing, and muscle strengthening, as well as the prevention of immobilization-related complications. Specifically, passive and assisted active mobility exercises of the hip, pelvis, and trunk are recommended as soon as the clinical condition allows, while monitoring fixation stability. For patients treated with ORIF alone, full weight-bearing is typically restricted for 6 to 12 weeks to protect bone healing, whereas in cases managed with combined procedures involving hip prosthesis (acute total hip arthroplasty), earlier loading may be permitted. Throughout rehabilitation, strengthening exercises targeting the gluteal muscles, quadriceps, and hip stabilizers should be included, together with gait training (using a cane or walker as required), balance exercises, and functional independence training in activities of daily living to minimize the risk of recurrent falls and promote functional recovery. Orthogeriatric coordination and management of comorbidities (osteoporosis, sarcopenia, nutrition) are also crucial to optimize outcomes. Overall, the lack of standardized protocols specifically designed for this elderly population necessitates individualized rehabilitation strategies according to fracture type, fixation quality, bone density, and the patient's pre-injury functional status [37, 38].

- Reoperations and satisfaction: A critical outcome aspect is whether treatment avoids or delays the need for further surgeries. As mentioned, primary arthroplasty appears to improve this aspect (fewer later conversions). Patient satisfaction in the elderly with surgery is also linked to achieving independent walking. Many reports indicate that, regardless of treatment, a significant proportion of patients over 65 require walking aids (cane or walker), even if pain relief is achieved. Specific hip functional outcome measures (HHS, Merle d'Aubigné) typically rate "good/excellent" in about 60–80% of cases that consolidate without severe arthritis, while cases with complications show low scores [1, 16, 18, 31–33, 36].

- Mortality and health status: From the perspective of global PROMs, it is important to note that high mortality acts as a "competing outcome." In combined series (~3,928 patients, mean age 72.6), cumulative mortality was about 21.6% at ~2 years, reflecting the frailty of these patients. Interestingly, mortality did not differ significantly between treatment types in adjusted analyses; thus, choosing surgery or not does not seem to affect survival in most cases, but rather depends on baseline condition. This underscores that PROMs and outcomes in survivors should be interpreted alongside the fact that about one-fifth do not survive follow-up, typically due to medical conditions [4, 15, 19].

In general, functional outcomes of acetabular fractures in patients over 65 years are modest. Surgical intervention (whether ORIF or arthroplasty) aims to improve pain control and allow early mobility but does not guarantee a return to full pre-injury physical capacity. Available PROMs indicate that, with an appropriate strategy for each patient, acceptable levels of function and quality of life can be achieved, with key goals being the prevention of chronic pain and hip stability. More prospective studies are needed to determine which treatment maximizes long-term PROMs, as current evidence is mostly retrospective and suggests no major difference in final quality of life between conservative and surgical management in comparable survivors. Therefore, therapeutic choice should be individualized, prioritizing the minimization of complications and the achievement of articular stability.

10. Conclusions

Over the last two decades, important knowledge has been accumulated to guide the management of acetabular fractures in patients over 65 years old:

- These injuries are increasing with the aging population, and despite often being low-energy fractures, they entail high morbidity and mortality (approximately 20% per year). A multidisciplinary approach is required, given the frailty of the elderly patient.

- The most common fracture patterns in the elderly involve the anterior column and the acetabular roof, with frequent bone impactions. The presence of comminution and dome impaction (the "gull sign") is a marker of poor prognosis for conventional reconstruction.

- Initial treatment includes temporary skeletal traction, medical optimization, and careful selection of the definitive strategy (conservative vs. surgical) based on the patient's condition and the fracture.

- Conservative management: valid in selected cases (stable fractures, inoperable patients), avoiding surgical risks but with the risk of functional limitation and late conversion to arthroplasty (~8%). It has the lowest rate of in-hospital medical complications, although intrinsic mortality remains high.

- ORIF (osteosynthesis) remains the cornerstone for restoring anatomy in displaced fractures. If an anatomic reduction is achieved, the best functional results are obtained. However, ORIF in the elderly has the highest postoperative complication and reoperation rates (up to ~20–30% require rescue arthroplasty), especially when acetabular dome impaction is present.

- Acute arthroplasty (combined THA) has emerged as an effective alternative in fractures with poor prognosis for ORIF. Comparative studies indicate that it reduces reoperations (fewer later conversions to THA) and offers functional results comparable to ORIF. This strategy is recommended for patients with risk factors for failure (comminuted dome, very advanced age, femoral damage). The use of dual mobility cups is advised to minimize dislocations.

- Late conversion to THA remains necessary in a relevant proportion of cases initially managed without a prosthesis. Conversion surgery is complex, but with appropriate techniques, it can relieve pain and improve function. Ideally, candidates for conversion are identified early to avoid delaying the inevitable.

- PROMs outcomes: There is no clear consensus on the superiority of one treatment over another in terms of patient-reported quality of life; differences are subtle and depend more on achieving pain-free stability than on the method itself. The priority is to individualize treatment, considering frailty, expectations, and fracture anatomy, aiming for maximum mobility with minimum pain and the fewest interventions.

In conclusion, the management of acetabular fractures in patients over 65 should be personalized and multidisciplinary. Options range from nonoperative management to internal fixation or acute arthroplasty, all carrying risks in this vulnerable population. Recent evidence points to modern strategies, such as fixation plus acute replacement, offering advantages in selected cases, while in others, a conservative approach remains valid. It is essential to continue gathering data (ideally via prospective studies or trials) to refine indications, but currently, the decision depends on balancing surgical risk, fracture pattern, and the likelihood of reconstruction success versus replacement.

Conflict of Interest

The authors declare no conflicts of interest.

Author details

Fernando Antunez-Muiños[1], Alberto Jorge-Mora[1,2*], Tamara de la Rasilla-Sainz[1], Belen Ines Vieira-Lopez[1], Diego Novillo-Casal[3], Jorge González-García[3], Felipe Ignacio Vergara-Gutiérrez[1] and Iván Castro-Arias[1]

1 Orthopedics and Trauma, Complexo Hospitalario of A Coruña, A Coruña, Spain

2 Musculoskeletal Pathology Group, IDIS, Santiago, Spain

3 Orthopedics and Trauma, Complexo Hospitalario of Santiago, Santiago de Compostela, Spain

*Address all correspondence to: aljmora@gmail.com

References

[1] Ferguson TA, Patel R, Bhandari M, Matta JM. Fractures of the acetabulum in patients aged 60 years and older: An epidemiological and radiological study. The Journal of Bone and Joint Surgery. British Volume. 2010; **92**(2):250–257

[2] Khalifa AA, Mahran DG, Fergany A, Farouk O. Epidemiology of acetabular fractures in elderly patients and the effect of various management options on the outcomes. A comprehensive narrative review. International Journal of Orthopaedic and Trauma Nursing. 2024;**53**:101049

[3] Simske N, Furdock R, Heimke I, Vallier HA. Acetabular fractures in elderly patients are associated with high rates of complications during the initial admission. Trauma Surgery & Acute Care Open. 2023;**8**(1):e001235

[4] Firoozabadi R, Cross WW, Krieg JC, Routt MLC. Acetabular fractures in the senior population- epidemiology, mortality and treatments. The Archives of Bone and Joint Surgery. 2017;**5**(2):96–102

[5] Krappinger D, Freude T, Stuby F, Lindtner RA. Acetabular fractures in geriatric patients: Epidemiology, pathomechanism, classification and treatment options. Archives of Orthopaedic and Trauma Surgery. 2024;**144**(10):4515–4524

[6] Cecil A, Yu JW, Rodriguez VA, Sima A, Torbert J, Satpathy J, et al. High- Versus low-energy acetabular fracture outcomes in the geriatric population. Geriatric Orthopaedic Surgery & Rehabilitation. 2020;**11**:2151459320939546

[7] Anglen JO, Burd TA, Hendricks KJ, Harrison P. The "Gull Sign": A harbinger of failure for internal fixation of geriatric acetabular fractures. Journal of Orthopaedic Trauma. 2003;**17** (9):625–634

[8] Lim EJ, Shon HC, Yang JY, Ahn J, Jj K, JW K. Surgical outcomes of acetabular fracture of elderly patients with superomedial dome impaction. Scientific Reports. 2023;**13**(1): 19091

[9] Parrino CR, Fransman RB, Varone AJ, Galvagno SM. Advanced trauma life support. In: Faintuch J, Faintuch S, editors. Recent Strategies in High Risk Surgery. Cham: Springer Nature Switzerland; 2024. p. 171–194

[10] Pj L, CY L, Tseng IC, Su CY, Hsu YH, Chou YC, et al. A retrospective study of Hip posterior fracture-dislocation: Closed reduction at the emergency department or in the operation theater? Journal of Orthopaedics and Traumatology. 2022;**23**:55

[11] Bumpass DB, Ricci WM, McAndrew CM, Gardner MJ. A prospective study of pain reduction and knee dysfunction comparing femoral skeletal traction and splinting in adult trauma patients. Journal of Orthopaedic Trauma. 2015;**29**(2): 112–118

[12] Nasuruddin H, Omar MS, Che Ahmad A, Bahaudin N, Ahmad Ismani MS. Radiological outcome of the gradual increase in skeletal traction in acetabular fracture. Cureus. 2025;**17**(1): e76725

[13] O'Toole RV, Stein DM, O'Hara NN, Frey KP, Taylor TJ, et al., Major Extremity Trauma Research C. Aspirin or low-molecular-weight heparin for thromboprophylaxis after a fracture. New England Journal of Medicine. 2023;**388**(3):203–213

[14] Keppler AM, Gosch M, Kammerlander C. Orthogeriatric co-management in pelvic and acetabular fractures. Archives of Orthopaedic and Trauma Surgery. 2024;**144**(10): 4595–4599

[15] Browner BD, Jupiter J, Krettek C, Anderson PA. Skeletal Trauma E-Book: Basic Science, Management, and Reconstruction, **2**. Elsevier Health Sciences; 2019

[16] Lannes X, Moerenhout K, Duong HP, Borens O, Steinmetz S. Outcomes of combined Hip procedure with dual mobility cup versus osteosynthesis for acetabular fractures in elderly patients: A retrospective observational cohort study of fifty one patients. International Orthopaedics. 2020;**44**(10):2131–2138

[17] Manson T, Schmidt AH. Acetabular fractures in the elderly: A critical analysis review. JBJS Reviews. 2016;**4**(10)

[18] Cacciola G, Aprato A, Branca Vergano L, Sallam A, Masse A. Is non-operative management of acetabular fracture a viable option for older patients? A systematic review of the literature for indication, treatments, complications and outcome. Acta Bio-medica : Atenei Parmensis. 2022;**92**(S3): e2021555

[19] McCormick BP, Serino J, Orman S, Webb AR, Wang DX, Mohamadi A, et al. Treatment modalities and outcomes following acetabular fractures in the elderly: A systematic review. European Journal of Orthopaedic Surgery & Traumatology. 2022;**32**: 649–659

[20] Riemenschneider J, Vollrath JT, Muhlenfeld N, Frank J, Marzi I, Janko M. Acetabular fractures treatment needs in the elderly and nonagenarians. EFORT Open Reviews. 2022;**7**(6): 433–445

[21] Zanna L, Ceri L, Scalici G, Boncinelli D, Burchette DT, Buzzi R, et al. Outcome of surgically treated acetabular fractures: Risk factors for postoperative complications and for early conversion to total Hip arthroplasty. European Journal of Orthopaedic Surgery & Traumatology. 2023;**33**:2419–2426

[22] Staresinic M, Lindtner RA, Krappinger D, Gansslen A. Posterior approaches to the acetabulum. Archives of Orthopaedic and Trauma Surgery. 2024;**144**(10):4633–4640

[23] Alton TB, Gee AO. Classifications in brief: Letournel classification for acetabular fractures. Clinical Orthopaedics and Related Research. 2014;**472**(1):35–38

[24] Das CP, Acharya MR, Makwana VR. Corrigendum to "Delayed presentation of complex acetabular fractures: Review of literature on outcome of internal fixations with reference to extended ilio-femoral approach" [J Clin Orthop Trauma 11(6) (2020) 1082-1089]. Journal of Clinical Orthopaedics and Trauma. 2021;**17**:282

[25] Griffin DB, Beaule PE, Matta JM. Safety and efficacy of the extended iliofemoral approach in the treatment of

complex fractures of the acetabulum. The Journal of Bone and Joint Surgery. British Volume. 2005;**87**(10):1391–1396

[26] Stockle U, Hoffmann R, Sudkamp NP, Reindl R, Haas NP. Treatment of complex acetabular fractures through a modified extended iliofemoral approach. Journal of Orthopaedic Trauma. 2002;**16**(4): 220–230

[27] Gemci C, Gultac E, Can FI, Sahin IG, Kilinc CY, Aydogan NH. Management of posterior wall acetabular fractures using the anterior intrapelvic approach with lag screw fixation: A retrospective clinical and radiological study. Medicine (Baltimore). 2025;**104**(41):e45060

[28] David G, Sagi CH, Guy P, Mauffrey C. Anterior intrapelvic approach: A comprehensive understanding of the anatomy. Journal of the American Academy of Orthopaedic Surgeons. 2025;**33** (19):1061–1070

[29] Brand A, von Ruden C, Probst C, Wenzel L, Augat P, Perl M. Early biomechanical outcome in patients with acetabular fractures treated using the pararectus approach: A gait and stair climb analysis study. European Journal of Trauma and Emergency Surgery. 2022;**48**(2):1307–1316

[30] Yao S, Chen K, Zhu F, Liu J, Wang Y, Zeng L, et al. Internal fixation of anterior acetabular fractures with a limited pararectus approach and the anatomical plates: Preliminary results. BMC Musculoskeletal Disorders. 2021;**22**:203

[31] Nicol GM, Sanders EB, Kim PR, Beaule PE, Gofton WT, Grammatopoulos G. Outcomes of total hip arthroplasty after acetabular open reduction and internal fixation in the elderly-acute vs delayed total hip arthroplasty. The Journal of Arthroplasty. 2021;**36**(2): 605–611

[32] Smakaj A, Rovere G, Scoscina D, De MD, Erasmo R, Battiato C, et al. Outcomes of acetabular fractures treated with acute fix and replace versus open reduction and internal fixation in elderly population: A multicentric retrospective study. International Orthopaedics. 2022;**46**:2659–2666

[33] Smakaj A, Rovere G, Battiato C, Erasmo R, De Mauro D, Fidanza A, et al. Mid-term outcomes of acetabular fractures treated with acute fix and replace versus ORIF in the elderly: A multicentric study with minimum 5-year follow-up. European Journal of Orthopaedic Surgery & Traumatology. 2025;**35**:192

[34] Aali Rezaie A, Blevins K, Kuo FC, Manrique J, Restrepo C, Parvizi J. Total hip arthroplasty after prior acetabular fracture: Infection is a real concern. The Journal of Arthroplasty. 2020;**35** (9):2619–2623

[35] Moon JK, Lee J, Yoon PW, Chang JS, Kim JW. Efficacy of total Hip arthroplasty after operatively treated acetabular fracture. Archives of Orthopaedic and Trauma Surgery. 2020;**140**(7):973–979

[36] Shaker F, Esmaeili S, Nakhjiri MT, Azarboo A, Shafiei SH. The outcome of conversion total Hip arthroplasty following acetabular fractures: A systematic review and meta-analysis of comparative studies. Journal of Orthopaedic Surgery and Research. 2024;**19**(1):83

[37] Samuel RAN, Prashanth KT, Thirunthaiyan MR, Kumar RD, Sundararaja B. Management of geriatric acetabulum fracture - A case report. Journal of Orthopaedic Case Reports. 2025;**15**(8):260–264

[38] Ivanova S, Prochazka O, Giannoudis PV, Tosounidis T, Tannast M, Bastian JD. Rehabilitation protocols for surgically treated acetabular fractures in older adults: Current practices and outcomes. Journal of Clinical Medicine. 2025;**14**(14)

Chapter 4

Spinal Fractures – Current Treatment Options and Perspectives

Slavisa Zagorac

Abstract

Spinal trauma is a complex injury that often requires a multidisciplinary approach and treatment. It is frequently associated with spinal cord injury and neurologic deficit. Spinal column injuries are most often caused by the action of a force of great intensity (traffic accidents, falls from a height, blows with a hard object) or the effect of a minor trauma (based on a previously altered vertebra, most often due to osteoporosis or tumor). This chapter will focus on providing a summary of steps in the initial evaluation of spinal trauma, spinal cord injuries, classification systems, and modern patterns of treatment.

Keywords: spinal trauma, spinal cord injuries, neurologic deficit, primary evaluation, modern treatment

1. Introduction

The spinal column consists of 33–34 vertebrae connected to each other by joints, ligaments, and muscles. Of these, 24 vertebrae are motile and are called true vertebrae (*vertebrae verae*) and include 7 cervical (*vertebrae cervicales*), 12 thoracic (*vertebrae thoracicae*), and 5 lumbar (*vertebrae lumbales*) vertebrae. In contrast, the sacral and coccygeal vertebrae are false vertebrae (*vertebrae spuriae*), which are fused together to form the sacrum (*os sacrum*) and the coccyx (*os coccyges*) [1–3]. The spinal vertebrae, connected to each other, form a spinal canal that extends along the entire length of the spinal column, and in this canal is located the spinal cord (*medulla spinalis*) with its sheaths – meninges, blood vessels, and the beginnings of spinal nerves (*nn. spinales*) [4, 5]. The spinal column is characterized by the increasing height of the vertebral bodies and disks from the cervical to the lumbar region. The largest width of the spinal column corresponds to the base of the sacrum because the entire weight of the upper body is transferred to the lower extremities through the joint of the sacrum with the pelvic bones [1, 2, 6].

The vertebra belongs to the type of short bones, irregular in shape. A typical vertebra has a body, an arch, a spinal opening, and seven processes [1, 7, 8].

There are four physiological curvatures in the spinal column. Thoracic kyphosis extends from Th2 to Th12, and sacral kyphosis extends from the lumbosacral articulation to the apex of the coccygeal bone. Cervical lordosis is formed when a newborn begins to raise its head [2, 9–11]. Lumbar lordosis extends from Th12 to the lumbosacral articulation [1, 2, 12]. With the activity of the erector spinae, which pulls the erect lumbar spine to achieve the position necessary for walking, lumbar lordosis is formed. Around the age of six, all four sagittal curves are definitively formed [13].

The movements that take place in the spinal column are movements of flexion, extension, lateral flexion, rotation, and circumduction. The intervertebral disks, as well as the facet articulations, allow and limit the movements of two adjacent vertebrae. The disks are thicker in the cervical and lumbar spine, so the movements in these regions are greater [1–3, 6].

2. Epidemiology of spinal column injuries

Spinal column injuries are characterized by a bimodal distribution: they are most common in younger people (from 15 to 30 years old) and in the elderly (over 65 years old). Injuries are most often caused by the action of a force of great intensity (traffic accidents, falls from a height, blows with a hard object) or the effect of a small trauma (based on a previously altered vertebra, most often due to osteoporosis or a tumor). In 10%–50% of cases of spinal column injury, neurological impairment occurs (quadriplegia or paraplegia) [14, 15].

The basic mechanisms of injury are defined by the direction and intensity of the force acting on the spinal column, and these are: flexion, extension, rotation, lateral flexion, compression (axial force), and distraction (stretching) [16–18].

3. Initial evaluation and management

Treatment of spinal cord injuries is based on three basic principles. The first step is initial prehospital treatment (stabilization and immobilization of the injured person), the second step is early hospital treatment (clinical examination, assessment of the neurological condition, diagnostics), and the third step is definitive treatment (conservative or surgical).

3.1 Clinical presentation and prehospital treatment of spinal column injuries – primary and secondary survey, and resuscitation

Spinal column injuries can manifest in a variety of ways, depending on which level is injured, which structure is affected, and to what extent. Most often, there is pain and spasm of the paravertebral musculature, and if there is an injury to the spinal cord, a neurological outburst may occur.

The first rule of initial treatment is to ensure vital functions, according to the ABCDE system (A-airway, B-breathing, C-circulation, D-disability, E-environment) [19–21].

After that, it is necessary to determine the possible existence of an injury to the spinal column. Any individual involved in a trauma is assumed to have cervical spine injuries until ruled out otherwise. So, the treatment of potential spinal injury begins at the accident scene with proper immobilization [22–25]. If the injured person is unconscious, always assume that there is an injury to the spinal column and then place an immobilization device – a rigid cervical collar or a firm spine board [26–28]. In sport-related injuries, the player's helmet or shoulder pads should be left in place until arrival at the hospital, where experienced personnel can remove them safely. Inadequate initial immobilization can contribute to further neurologic deterioration in a patient with an acute SCI and worsen the outcome [22, 29].

If the injured person is conscious, make eye contact and ask them if they have pain in the cervical or thoracolumbar spine, if they can move their head, and if they have preserved movement and sensation in their arms and legs. If there is any confirmation of these symptoms, assume that there is a spinal injury and immediately apply immobilization. What is important is that the immediate absence of signs of neurological failure does not eliminate the possibility of spinal cord injury [30–33].

Polytraumatized patients should undergo a visual and manual inspection of the back. Motorcyclists are more likely to sustain thoracic spinal injuries. Flexion-distraction injuries should be suspected in the setting of abdominal ecchymoses or abrasions from a seat belt [17].

3.2 Early inpatient treatment – clinical examination, assessment of neurological status, diagnostics

After the initial treatment and ensuring vital functions, it is necessary to carefully take an anamnesis (data on the mechanism of injury) and conduct a clinical examination. If the patient is conscious and there is an injury to the spinal column, the injured person will complain of pain in the area of the injury. If there is also a neurological deficit, the injured person will complain of numbness, weakness in the arms and legs, or complete anesthesia from the level of the injury, as well as urinary retention [30–32].

Then a clinical examination is performed, which involves turning the injured person on their side (with the help of three people, where one simultaneously turns the head of the injured, another the torso, and the third the legs), followed by an inspection (to notice any deformity or the existence of abrasions or bruises), and then performing palpation to identify painful sensitivity and deformity [25].

This is followed by a detailed assessment of the neurological condition of the injured person, which is crucial for further treatment in the case of spinal injury. A neurological examination should include an assessment of muscle strength, sensitivity, and deep reflexes in the upper and lower extremities. A neurological status assessment protocol called the American Spinal Injury Association Score (ASIA score) has been introduced [34] (see **Figure 1**).

Cervical spine clearance in trauma patients remains controversial. Prolonged immobilization in polytrauma patients is known to be associated with numerous complications, including increased risk of aspiration, limitation of respiratory function, development of ulcers in the occipital and mandibular areas, and an increase in intracranial pressure [26, 27, 29].

Injuries can be ruled out via the National Emergency X-radiography Utilization Study (NEXUS) or Canadian Cervical Spine Rule (CCR) criteria in asymptomatic patients [35, 36] (see **Figures 2** and **3**).

After initial stabilization, ATLS (Advanced Trauma Life Support) measures, and clinical examination, diagnostics follow:

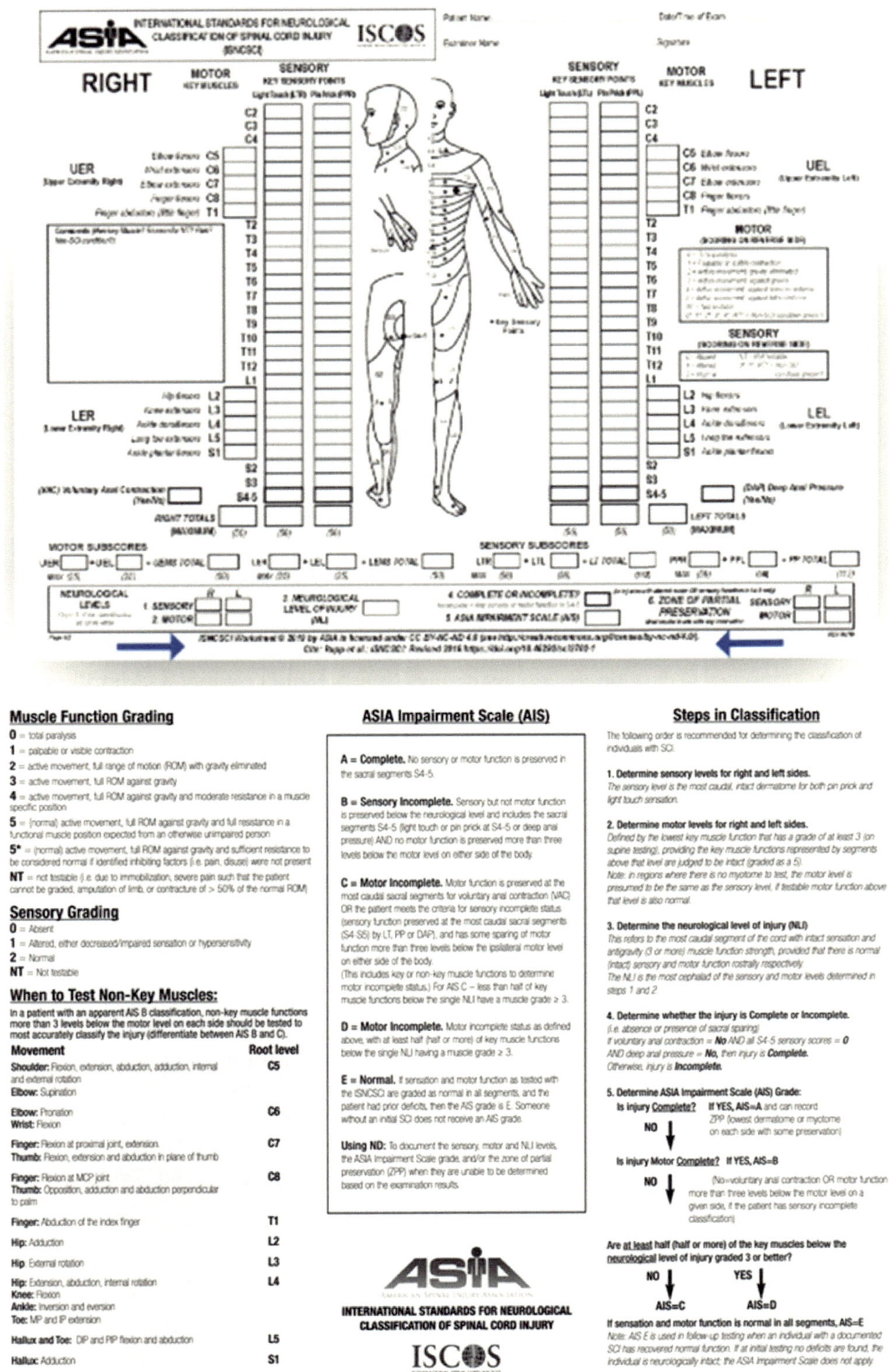

ASIA
INTERNATIONAL STANDARDS FOR NEUROLOGICAL CLASSIFICATION OF SPINAL CORD INJURY (ISNCSCI)
ISCOS

RIGHT — MOTOR KEY MUSCLES — SENSORY KEY SENSORY POINTS

SENSORY KEY SENSORY POINTS — MOTOR KEY MUSCLES — LEFT

UER (Upper Extremity Right): C5, C6, C7, C8, T1

UEL (Upper Extremity Left): C5, C6, C7, C8, T1

C2, C3, C4, T2, T3, T4, T5, T6, T7, T8, T9, T10, T11, T12, L1

LER (Lower Extremity Right): L2, L3, L4, L5, S1

LEL (Lower Extremity Left): L2, L3, L4, L5, S1

S2, S3, S4-5

MOTOR

SENSORY

RIGHT TOTALS (MAXIMUM)

LEFT TOTALS (MAXIMUM)

MOTOR SUBSCORES

SENSORY SUBSCORES

NEUROLOGICAL LEVELS — 1. SENSORY — 2. MOTOR

3. NEUROLOGICAL LEVEL OF INJURY (NLI)

4. COMPLETE OR INCOMPLETE?

5. ASIA IMPAIRMENT SCALE (AIS)

6. ZONE OF PARTIAL PRESERVATION — SENSORY — MOTOR

Muscle Function Grading

0 = total paralysis

1 = palpable or visible contraction

2 = active movement, full range of motion (ROM) with gravity eliminated

3 = active movement, full ROM against gravity

4 = active movement, full ROM against gravity and moderate resistance in a muscle specific position

5 = (normal) active movement, full ROM against gravity and full resistance in a functional muscle position expected from an otherwise unimpaired person

5* = (normal) active movement, full ROM against gravity and sufficient resistance to be considered normal if identified inhibiting factors (i.e. pain, disuse) were not present

NT = not testable (i.e. due to immobilization, severe pain such that the patient cannot be graded, amputation of limb, or contracture of > 50% of the normal ROM)

Sensory Grading

0 = Absent

1 = Altered, either decreased/impaired sensation or hypersensitivity

2 = Normal

NT = Not testable

When to Test Non-Key Muscles:

In a patient with an apparent AIS B classification, non-key muscle functions more than 3 levels below the motor level on each side should be tested to most accurately classify the injury (differentiate between AIS B and C).

Movement	Root level
Shoulder: Flexion, extension, abduction, adduction, internal and external rotation **Elbow:** Supination	C5
Elbow: Pronation **Wrist:** Flexion	C6
Finger: Flexion at proximal joint, extension. **Thumb:** Flexion, extension and abduction in plane of thumb	C7
Finger: Flexion at MCP joint **Thumb:** Opposition, adduction and abduction perpendicular to palm	C8
Finger: Abduction of the index finger	T1
Hip: Adduction	L2
Hip: External rotation	L3
Hip: Extension, abduction, internal rotation **Knee:** Flexion **Ankle:** Inversion and eversion **Toe:** MP and IP extension	L4
Hallux and Toe: DIP and PIP flexion and abduction	L5
Hallux: Adduction	S1

ASIA Impairment Scale (AIS)

A = Complete. No sensory or motor function is preserved in the sacral segments S4-5.

B = Sensory Incomplete. Sensory but not motor function is preserved below the neurological level and includes the sacral segments S4-5 (light touch or pin prick at S4-5 or deep anal pressure) AND no motor function is preserved more than three levels below the motor level on either side of the body.

C = Motor Incomplete. Motor function is preserved at the most caudal sacral segments for voluntary anal contraction (VAC) OR the patient meets the criteria for sensory incomplete status (sensory function preserved at the most caudal sacral segments (S4-S5) by LT, PP or DAP), and has some sparing of motor function more than three levels below the ipsilateral motor level on either side of the body.
(This includes key or non-key muscle functions to determine motor incomplete status.) For AIS C – less than half of key muscle functions below the single NLI have a muscle grade ≥ 3.

D = Motor Incomplete. Motor incomplete status as defined above, with at least half (half or more) of key muscle functions below the single NLI having a muscle grade ≥ 3.

E = Normal. If sensation and motor function as tested with the ISNCSCI are graded as normal in all segments, and the patient had prior deficits, then the AIS grade is E. Someone without an initial SCI does not receive an AIS grade.

Using ND: To document the sensory, motor and NLI levels, the ASIA Impairment Scale grade, and/or the zone of partial preservation (ZPP) when they are unable to be determined based on the examination results.

ASIA
AMERICAN SPINAL INJURY ASSOCIATION
INTERNATIONAL STANDARDS FOR NEUROLOGICAL CLASSIFICATION OF SPINAL CORD INJURY
ISCOS

Steps in Classification

The following order is recommended for determining the classification of individuals with SCI.

1. Determine sensory levels for right and left sides.
The sensory level is the most caudal, intact dermatome for both pin prick and light touch sensation.

2. Determine motor levels for right and left sides.
Defined by the lowest key muscle function that has a grade of at least 3 (on supine testing), providing the key muscle functions represented by segments above that level are judged to be intact (graded as a 5).
Note: in regions where there is no myotome to test, the motor level is presumed to be the same as the sensory level, if testable motor function above that level is also normal.

3. Determine the neurological level of injury (NLI)
This refers to the most caudal segment of the cord with intact sensation and antigravity (3 or more) muscle function strength, provided that there is normal (intact) sensory and motor function rostrally respectively.
The NLI is the most cephalad of the sensory and motor levels determined in steps 1 and 2.

4. Determine whether the injury is Complete or Incomplete.
(i.e. absence or presence of sacral sparing)
If voluntary anal contraction = ***No*** *AND all S4-5 sensory scores =* ***0***
AND deep anal pressure = ***No****, then injury is* ***Complete.***
Otherwise, injury is ***Incomplete.***

5. Determine ASIA Impairment Scale (AIS) Grade:

Is injury Complete? **If YES, AIS=A** and can record ZPP (lowest dermatome or myotome on each side with some preservation)

NO ↓

Is injury Motor Complete? **If YES, AIS=B**

NO ↓ (No=voluntary anal contraction OR motor function more than three levels below the motor level on a given side, if the patient has sensory incomplete classification)

Are at least half (half or more) of the key muscles below the neurological level of injury graded 3 or better?

NO ↓ **AIS=C** **YES** ↓ **AIS=D**

If sensation and motor function is normal in all segments, AIS=E
Note: AIS E is used in follow-up testing when an individual with a documented SCI has recovered normal function. If at initial testing no deficits are found, the individual is neurologically intact; the ASIA Impairment Scale does not apply.

Figure 1.
ASIA Standard Neurological Classification of Spinal Cord Injury (from International Standards for Neurological Classification of Spinal Cord Injury). (Reproduced with permission from http://asia-spinalinjury.org.).

DOI: http://dx.doi.org/10.5772/intechopen.1014132

Nexus Criteria

In the NEXUS study, a clinical clearance protocol consisting of five criteria was validated with a 100% sensitivity for the exclusion of cervical spinal injury.
Protocol:

1st - assess signs of intoxication in the patient.
2nd - assess for the presence of focal neurologic deficits.
3rd - assessment for the presence of painful distracting injuries.
4th - assess whether the patient has a normal level of alertness.
5th - presence of posterior midline tenderness to palpation.

If no painful response is elicited and the patient has met all prior criteria, the C-collar can be removed and C-spine imaging is not needed.

Figure 2.
NEXUS criteria for c-spine injury.

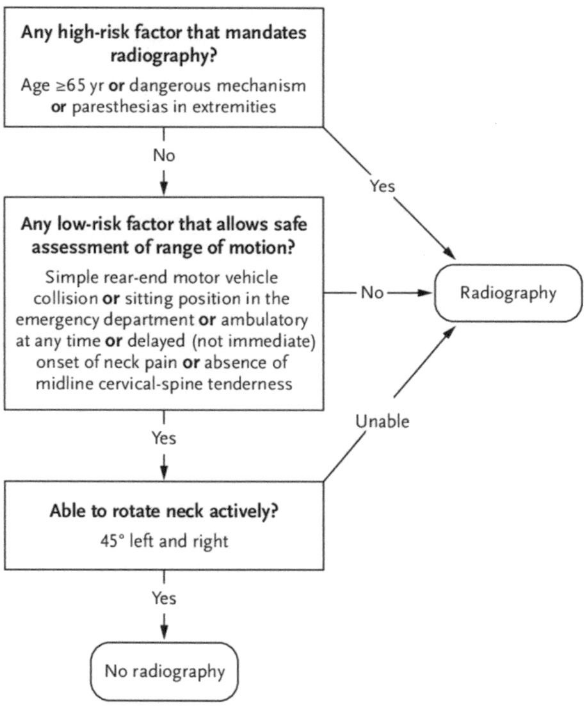

Figure 3.
The Canadian C-spine rule diagram.

(1) Conventional radiography – In a stable patient with a suspected spinal injury, it is necessary to perform an AP image, a profile (the most important, as it detects up to 80% of injuries), and, in the case of a suspected cervical spine injury, an additional image of the odontoid through the mouth and optionally two oblique shots. Adequate radiography involves visualizing all seven cervical vertebrae, including the first thoracic vertebra. If the patient is conscious, there are two important algorithms based on which we assess whether the injured person needs radiographs, that is, when we are sure that there is no serious injury to the

cervical spine (previously mentioned: the NEXUS criteria and the Canadian C-Spine Rule; see **Figures 4–7**).

(2) Computed tomography – CT scan – It is today the gold standard in the evaluation of bone-articular injuries of the spine in a polytraumatized or unconscious injured person, as well as in cases where radiographs are not usable. A CT scan of the whole body is often performed as part of the trauma protocol. Modern CT machines enable 3D and dynamic reconstruction of the injured segment. If the clinical findings are normal and the radiography is adequate, a CT scan should be avoided due to the high dose of radiation (see **Figure 8–10**)

(3) Nuclear magnetic resonance imaging (NMR) – It is indicated in cases where there is a neurological deficit, and radiographs and CT scans are normal. It is invaluable in the detection of soft tissue injuries, in the suspicion of traumatic herniation of the disk (especially if there is a dislocation of the vertebrae), and in the suspicion of the existence of hematomas (see **Figure 11**).

(4) Myelography – Nowadays, it is rarely performed. It involves the injection of a contrast agent into the spinal canal, followed by an X-ray or CT scan. It is indicated in cases where there is a suspicion of intradural or epidural pathology (such as traumatic disk herniation or hematoma) and in cases where NMR is contraindicated.

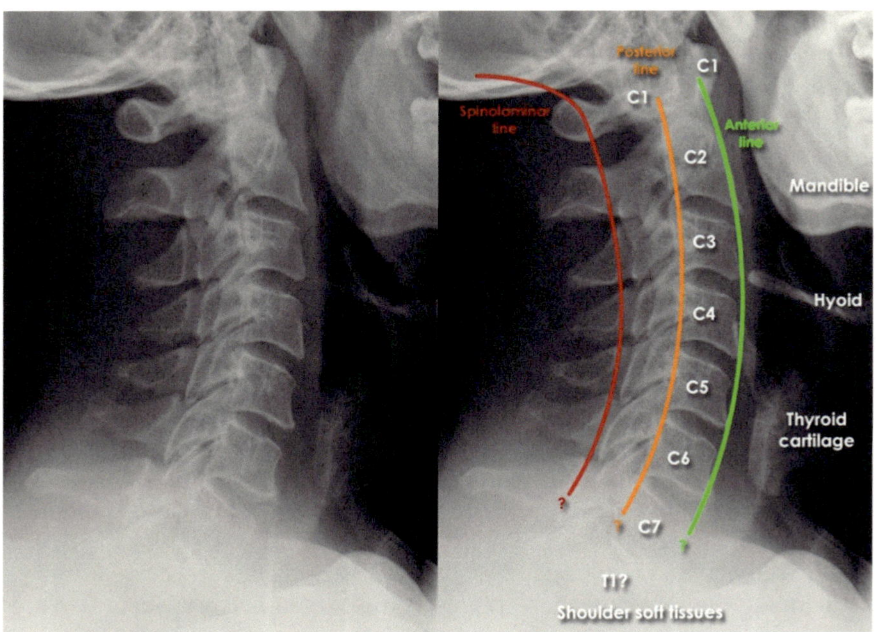

Figure 4.
Normal x ray of the cervical spine – lateral view (reproduced with permission from www.radiologymasterclass.co.uk).

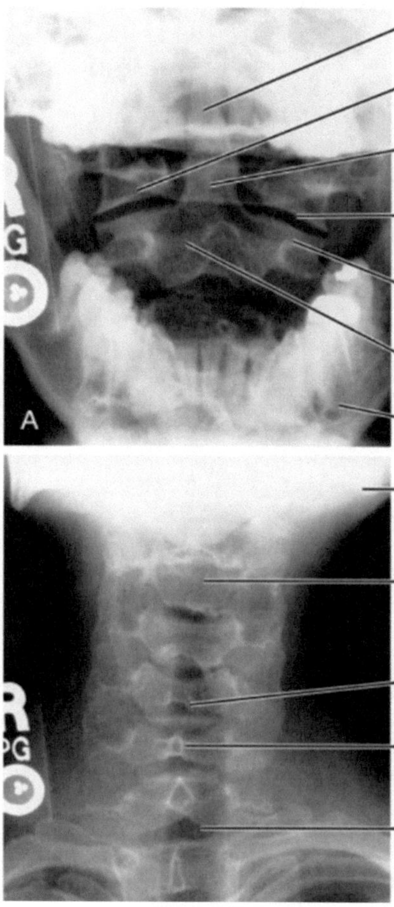

Figure 5.
AP odontoid view from the study by Mettler FA: Essentials of Radiology.

(5) Electromyeloneurography – EMNG – This method is important for monitoring the neurological recovery of the injured person and is not valid in the first weeks following the injury.

3.3 Definitive treatment (conservative or surgical) – the principles of modern treatment and surgical techniques

It is important to determine whether it is a stable or unstable fracture. Stable (minor) fractures without neurological deficit are treated conservatively by administering analgesics, wearing appropriate immobilization (neck: Philadelphia collar for 6 to 12 weeks, TLS orthosis for 12 weeks), and regular monitoring of the injured person. If it is an unstable injury, then surgical treatment is indicated, which has two goals: stabilization of the spinal column and decompression of the spinal canal [37–39].

Skeletal traction of the cervical spine (Crutchfield skull traction) is a very common procedure in the initial treatment of injuries to the cervical spine, especially dislocations [40, 41]. With the help of traction, first of all, further displacement of

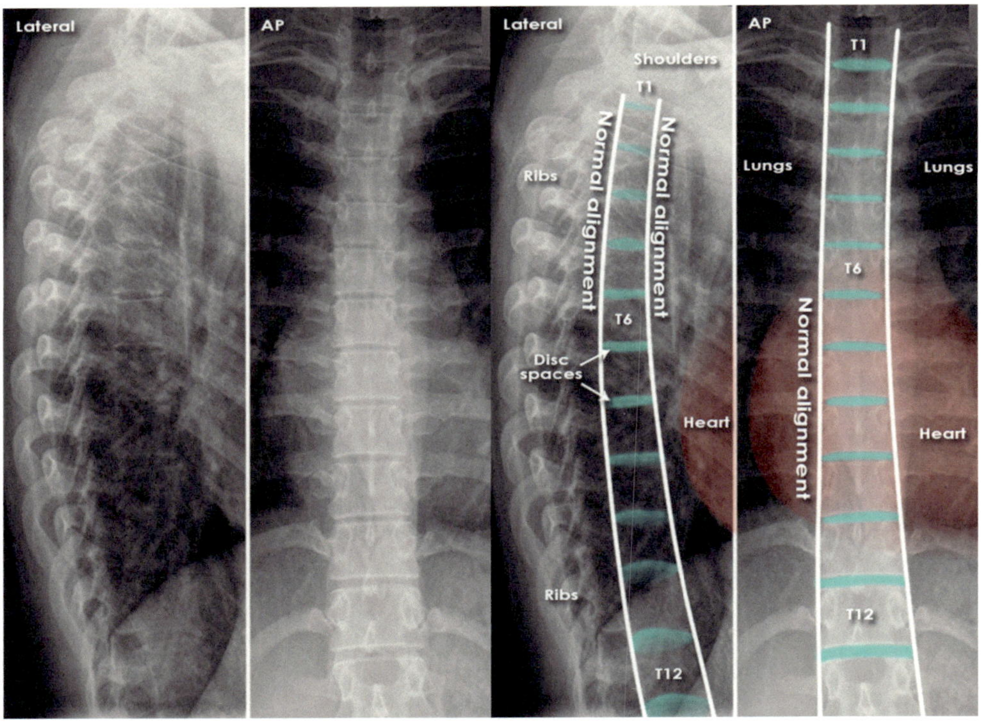

Figure 6.
Normal x ray of the thoracic spine – AP and lateral view (reproduced with permission from www.radiologymasterclass.co.uk).

the vertebrae is prevented, which would lead to a deterioration of the neurological status. In addition, with this method, a closed reposition can sometimes be achieved with a special maneuver. Skeletal traction placement technique: skeletal traction is placed under conditions of local anesthesia. Then, a small incision is made with a scalpel 1 cm above the earlobe. A pair of pliers is used to enter the tabula externa as much as 1 mm. Weights of a certain amount are then hung (a rough rule is to add a minimum of 2 kg to the injured segment. Example: if the C4 is luxated, then the load is 4 + 2 kg, a total of 6 kg).

The type of surgical treatment depends on the type of injury. If it is an unstable fracture, stabilization of this segment is indicated, which is achieved by using special screws and inserts that are usually made of titanium. In addition to stabilizing the fracture, decompression is necessary – relieving the spinal cord or nerve from pressure, which is achieved by removing a bone fragment or hematoma that leads to compression and, therefore, to a neurological deficit. This is done using one of the following techniques: corpectomy, laminectomy, laminoplasty, foraminotomy, or diskectomy.

Standard indications for the surgical treatment of thoracolumbar fractures include incomplete neurological deficit, progressive neurological deficit, spinal cord compression, fracture with luxation, kyphosis greater than 30 degrees, and associated injuries requiring early mobilization [42–44].

Modern spinal surgery involves two basic principles: classical and minimally invasive surgery. Whenever possible (depending primarily on the indication), the

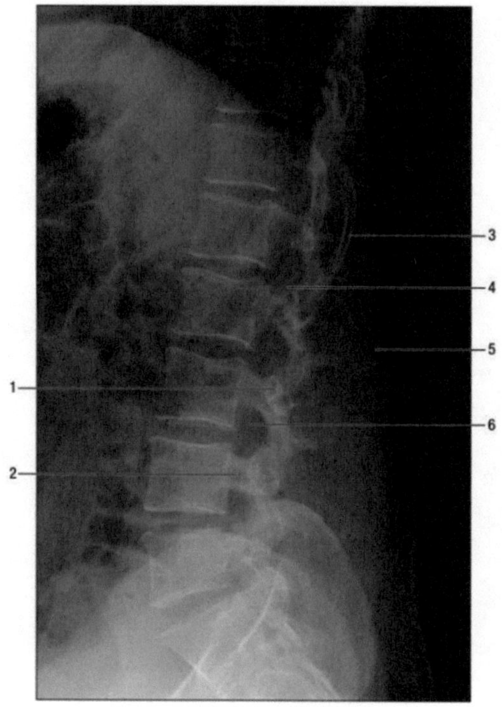

Figure 7.
Normal X ray of the lumbosacral spine – lateral view (from Standring S. Gray's Anatomy: The Anatomical Basis of Clinical practice. 41st ed. Philadelphia, PA: Elsevier; 2016. Fig. 43.44).

principles of minimally invasive surgery should be applied, as it aims at minimal trauma for the injured and faster postoperative recovery. Today's minimally invasive surgery for spinal cord injuries includes percutaneous placement of screws (with the help of X-rays or navigation), strengthening (augmentation) of the vertebrae with special bone cement, and thoracoscopically assisted decompression and fixation of the thoracic part of the spinal column [45–48].

There are three basic approaches: back (the most common), front, and combined front-back approach. Which approach will be used depends on the type of fracture, the existence of comorbidities and associated injuries, and the training of the surgeon.

3.3.1 Surgical approaches in injuries of the cervical spine

In the case of injuries to the cervical spine, the anterior approach is most often used. The anterior approach allows visualization of the subaxial cervical spine (C3–C7). Indications for the anterior approach include excision of the traumatic disk hernia, intervertebral fusion, tumor treatment, stabilization of a possible pathological fracture, stabilization of the traumatic fracture, and decompression of the spinal canal. The patient is positioned in supination, with the head in extension and facing the opposite side of the planned incision. The incision can be made on either the left or right side of the neck and can be transverse (from the midline of the neck to the anterior edge of the *m. sternocleidomastoideus*) or longitudinal (along the

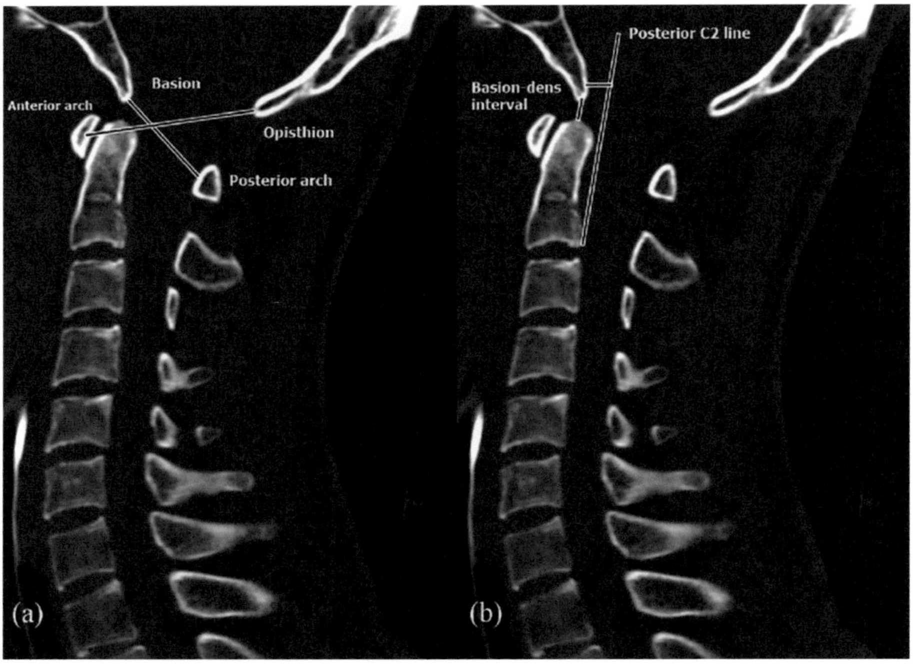

Figure 8.
Cervical spine CT scan with normal findings: (a) Power's ratio and (b) Basion-dens interval and Harris method. (Available from: https://www.researchgate.net/figure/cervical-spine-ct-scan-with-normal-findings-a-powers-ratio-and-b-basion-dens_fig2340020462 [accessed 7 Sept 2025]).

anterior edge of the same muscle). During anterior access to the neck, the most important structure at risk of injury is the *n. laryngeus recurrens*. Due to the specific anatomy of the right and left *n. laryngeus recurrens*, an incision is usually made on the left side because the right nerve is more exposed to injury [49–51].

The posterior approach allows visualization, in addition to the subaxial cervical spine, of C1 and C2, which cannot be accessed through the front of the neck. Indications for this approach include stabilization of fractures of C1 and C2, decompression of the spinal canal, intervertebral fusion, and treatment of tumors. The patient is positioned prone, with their head in flexion. The incision extends from the central prominence of the occipital bone (*protuberantia occipitalis*) down the midline for 6 to 8 cm. With this approach, injury to the occipital nerves and the vertebral artery (*a. vertebralis)* is possible [49, 52].

3.3.2 Surgical approaches in injuries of the thoracolumbar spine

The posterior approach is the most common form of surgical treatment for thoracolumbar spine injuries. In addition to providing access to the *cauda equina* and intervertebral disks, it can also reveal the posterior elements of the spinal column: spinous processes, laminae, facet joints, and pedicles. Access is through the midline and can be extended proximally and distally. The indications are as follows: excision of the traumatic disk hernia, intervertebral fusion, treatment of tumors, stabilization of a possible pathological fracture, stabilization of the traumatic fracture, and decompression of the spinal canal. The patient is in a prone position. Supports are

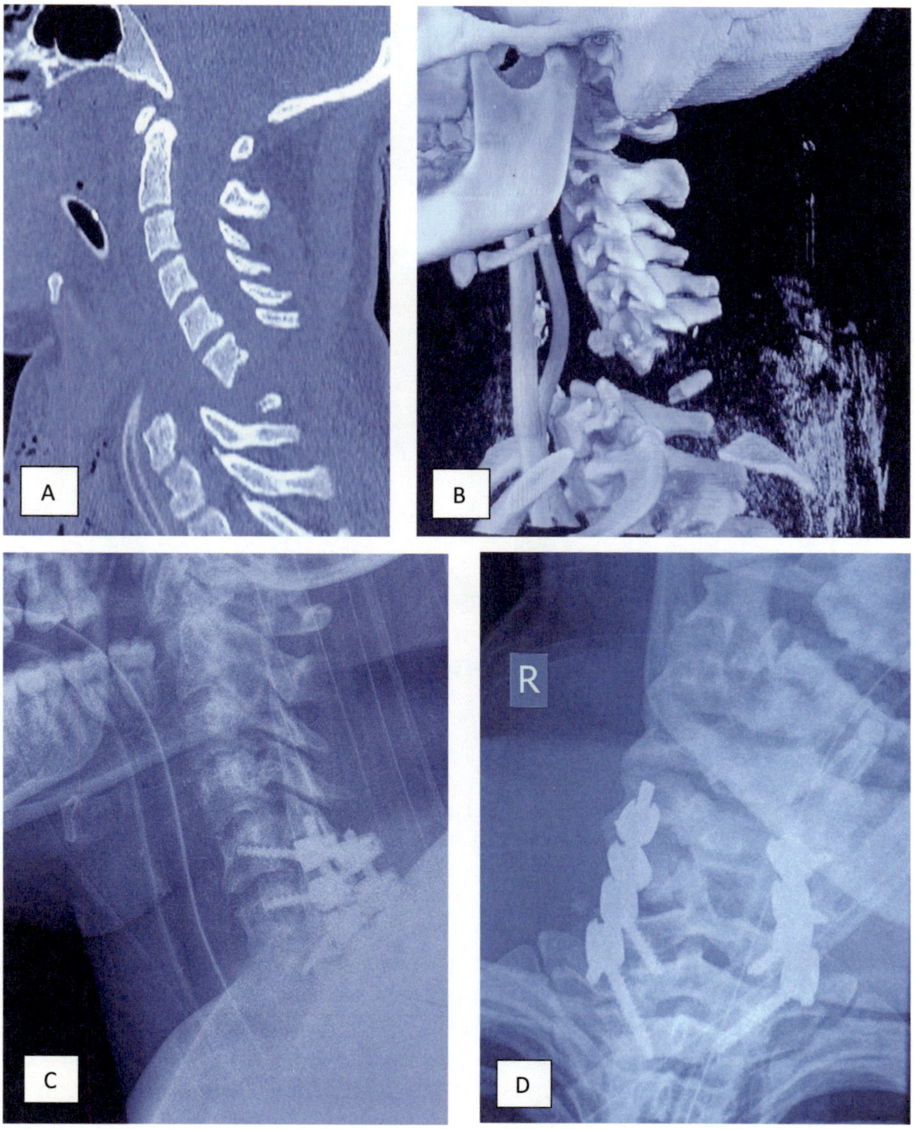

Figure 9.
A 19-year-old woman sustained a C6–C7 injury in a motor vehicle accident. (a) and (b) Show a CT scan of a completely dislocated vertebra. The ASIA score was A, and after surgery, the patient was moving her left arm. (c) and (d) Show RTG postoperatively with fixation of the C5, C6, C7, and Th1.

placed longitudinally under the chest, hips, and legs. Underneath the chest and hips, struts are placed to allow the abdomen to be completely free, reducing the filling of the venous plexus around the spinal cord and allowing the venous plexus to drain directly into the inferior vena cava. The patient's shoulders are positioned at an angle of no more than 90 degrees of abduction and should be slightly bent forward to relax the *plexus brachialis*. The head and neck are placed in a relaxed, neutral position, without pressure on the eyes. Avoid keeping the head lower than the rest of the body to reduce the risk of postoperative blindness (due to the high hydrostatic pressure in the eyes leading to reduced perfusion). If the approach is used for decompression, the hips are

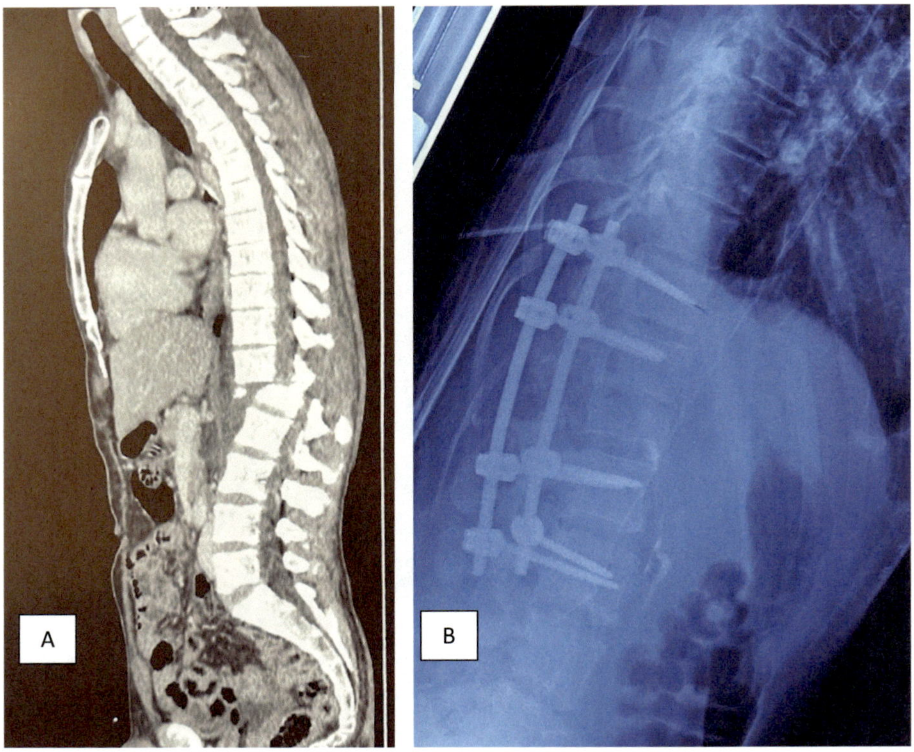

Figure 10.
A 34-year-old man sustained a fracture of the L1 vertebra with dislocation in a motor vehicle accident. (a) Shows CT scan after injury. (b) Shows RTG postoperatively with fixation of Th11, Th12, L2 and L3. The patient was paraplegic.

bent to increase the interlaminar or interspinous distance. By placing a brace under the ankle joint, the knees are bent without putting pressure on the proximal fibula-region of the common peroneal nerve [49, 53–56].

In addition to the posterior–posterior access, the thoracic spine can be accessed anteriorly (transthoracically) and postero-laterally, and the lumbar spine can be accessed anteriorly (transperitoneal and retroperitoneal) and posterolaterally (retroperitoneal) [49].

3.3.3 Minimally invasive stabilization of spinal fractures

Minimally invasive surgery is a modern approach to the treatment of spinal fractures, which is based on a well-established indication, a good choice of patients, and the necessity of special equipment. This implies the presence of a C-arc (movable X-ray machine) and the existence of a special instrument for placing screws. Sometimes, it is necessary to have neuromonitoring in order to monitor neurological functions during surgery, and lately, it has been used in more equipped centers for navigation. The concept of minimally invasive surgery involves minimal incision in the skin and minimal damage to subcutaneous tissue, muscles, and bone tissue. If it is a last resort, special needles and AP and profile X-rays are used to identify the target vertebrae. After that, special screws are

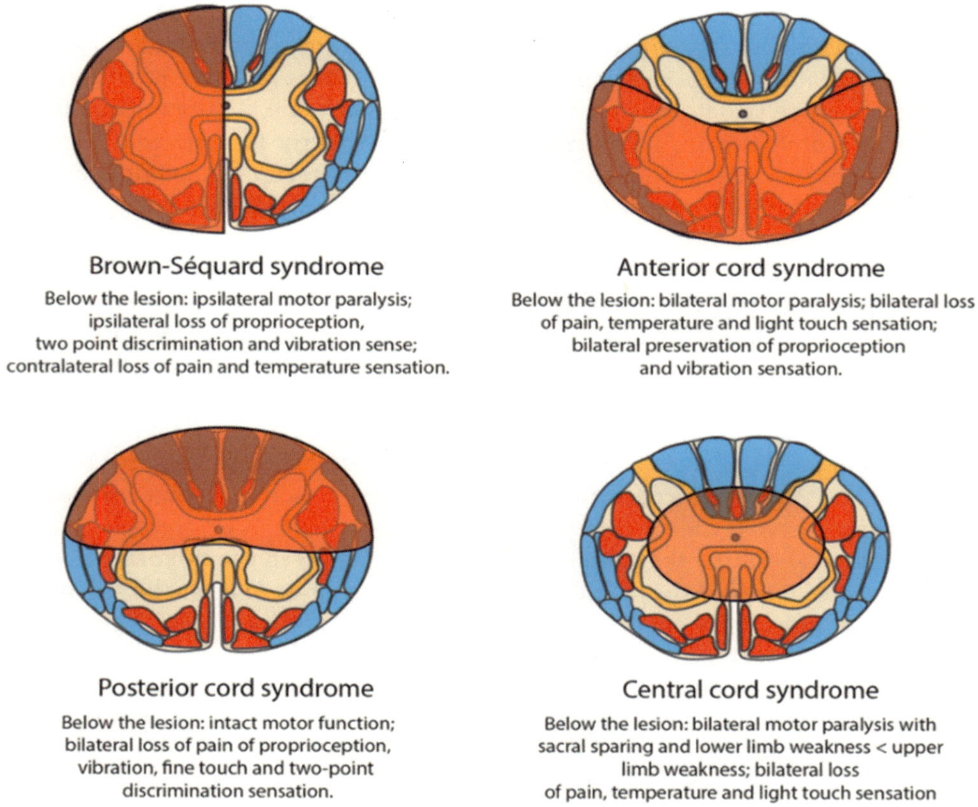

Figure 11.
Incomplete spinal cord lesions.

placed over these needles, which are perforated (hollow) in the middle so that they can be placed over the previously placed needles. After X-ray confirmation of the good position of the screws, two rods are placed over two additional small cuts to connect the screws. In most minimally invasive surgery systems, there is also the possibility of placing bone cement through screws with the aim of further strengthening the vertebrae, and this is especially important in cases of osteoporosis or metastasis [46, 49].

4. Spinal cord injuries

4.1 Background

The spinal cord is the caudal part of the central nervous system and lies entirely in the spinal canal (*canalis vertebralis*). It extends rostrally to the upper edge of the anterior arch of the atlas, where it continues to the medulla (medulla oblongata) and ends caudally at the L2 level. It has the shape of an elongated cylinder, 42–45 cm long. The terminal part of the spinal cord, 1–2 cm long, is called the *conus medullaris*. From the top of the cone starts the final thread (*filum terminale*). The spinal cord is made up of gray and white matter. The gray matter is made up of nerve cell bodies, dendrites, and glial cells. White matter is a set of axons and dendrites (myelinated nerve tract fibers, unmyelinated axons, and glial cells). The spinal cord is enveloped by three sheaths that separate it from the bone-connective structures of the walls of the spinal canal: on the outside is the dura mater, on the inside is the arachnoidea, and directly adjacent to the spinal cord is the soft membrane (pia mater). The space between the arachnoid and the pia mater is referred to as the subarachnoid space, which is filled with cerebrospinal fluid [4, 5, 57, 58].

The spinal cord has 31 pairs of spinal nerves. These are 8 cervical, 12 thoracic, 5 lumbar, 5 sacral, and 1 coccygeal. Spinal nerves exit the spinal canal through the intervertebral openings (*foramen intervertebrale*). Due to the unevenness in the length of the spinal cord and the spinal canal, the spinal nerves starting from the lumbar and sacral segments are almost parallel to the spinal cord, surround the cone, and form the final bundle of nerves – the *cauda equina* [57]. Each spinal nerve has an anterior and posterior root. The surface of the skin innervated by sensitive fibers of one spinal nerve is called a dermatome. The portion of muscle mass that corresponds to one spinal nerve is called the myotome.

The blood supply to the spinal cord is quite poor, given the importance of this tissue. Ischemia of the spinal cord can easily occur even after the slightest injury. Ischemia is particularly common at the levels of Th4 and L1. The arterial blood vessels of the spinal cord originate from the vertebral arteries (*aa. vertebrales*) and from the segmental arteries (*a. cervicalis profunda, a. cervicalis ascendens, a. intercostales posteriores, a. lumbales, a. iliolumbalis, a. sacrales laterales*) [5].

The annual incidence of SCI is approximately 17,700 new cases per year. Motor vehicle accidents and falls together are responsible for 69.9% of SCI, with gunshot wounds accounting for 13.8% and sports injuries for 8.2%. Fifty-four percent of SCI injuries occur in the cervical spine. Neurologically, most patients (45.8%) sustain incomplete quadriplegia, followed by incomplete paraplegia (21%), complete paraplegia (20%), and complete quadriplegia (17.5%) [4, 57].

4.2 Spinal cord injuries

Spinal cord injuries can be complete or incomplete. A complete lesion implies a complete loss of function below the level of injury. It is manifested by flaccid paralysis (atony), loss of reflexes (areflexia), flexed elbows, vasomotor paralysis with hypotension, hypothermia, bradycardia, priapism (parasympathetic paralysis), and, if the injury is above C4, the diaphragm is compromised, so patients with this level of injury most likely require intubation.

4.2.1 Incomplete lesions of the spinal cord are

(1) "Central cord" syndrome, which occurs in hyperextension injuries of the cervical spine in individuals with pre-existing stenosis of the spinal canal, is manifested by greater motor damage to the upper extremities than to the lower extremities [59–61]; (see **Figure 12**).

(2) "Anterior cord" syndrome, which has a vascular etiology and is manifested by loss of motor skills, sense of pain, and temperature; this injury carries

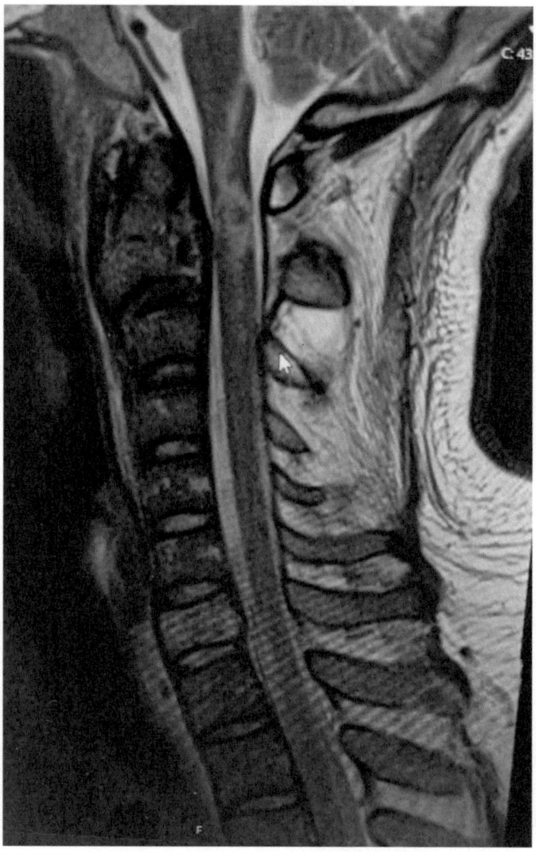

Figure 12.
A 23-year-old man sustained an injury to the cervical spine during diving. He suffered a C2 fracture with neurologic deficit (ASIA score was A). NMR at T2 sequence shows a spinal cord lesion at the level of the second cervical vertebra. After surgery, the patient recovered well enough to be reclassified as an ASIA D within nine months.

the worst prognosis of incomplete injuries, with only 10% to 20% of patients recovering functional motor control [59, 62, 63] (see **Figure 12**)

(3) "Brown-Séquard" syndrome, which occurs due to lateral hemisection of the spinal cord in penetrating injuries, is manifested by ipsilateral hemiparesis and loss of deep and vibrational sensitivity, as well as contralateral loss of pain and temperature. This injury carries the best prognosis for recovery of functional motor activity and sphincter control [59, 64, 65] (see **Figure 12**)

(4) "Posterior cord" syndrome is a rare, incomplete spinal cord injury that selectively affects the posterior (dorsal) columns, leading to a loss of proprioception (body position sense) and vibration sense, as well as an ataxic gait [59, 66] (see **Figure 12**).

Early neurological findings may be confounded by spinal shock, which is a reversible functional impairment of the spinal cord. As a result of spinal shock, there is a temporary inhibition of the reflex functions of the spinal cord. At the stage of spinal shock, there is flaccid paralysis, loss of reflexes, loss of all modalities of sensation, urinary retention, distension of the intestine with constipation, and vasomotor paralysis with hypotension and hypothermia. This phase can last 24–72 hours, and sometimes longer. After exiting the phase of spinal shock, the sign of recovery is the induction of the bulbocavernosus reflex [59, 67, 68].

4.2.2 Treatment of acute spinal cord injury

It must be carried out within eight hours of the onset of the injury, and preferably within the first three hours, in order to improve post-injury outcomes and prevent secondary spinal cord damage.

(1) Neuroprotective and pharmacological strategies – NASCIS III protocol
Specific therapy involves the administration of methylprednisolone intravenously at an initial dose of 30 mg/kg bolus, followed by an intravenous infusion of 5.4 mg/(kg h) for the next 23 hours. For patients presenting 3 to 8 hours after injury, the 30 mg/kg bolus is followed by 5.4 mg/(kg h) for the next 47 hours [69].

(2) Surgical management
The Surgical Timing in Acute Spinal Cord Injury Study (STASCIS) recommends spinal cord decompression within 24 hours in patients with SCI. This early decompression results in an increase of a two-grade ASIA impairment score improvement [70].

5. Cervical fractures

5.1 Classification of injuries of the cervical spine

The most recent classification that has found application in clinical practice is the AO Spine Injury Classification System, which provides a specific classification of injuries of the upper (C1–C2) and subaxial cervical spine (C3–C7), and also includes the neurological condition of the patient [71, 72] (see **Figure 13**).

5.1.1 Occipital condyle fractures

Incidence is 3% to 16%. Typical clinical presentation can include high cervical pain, torticollis, headaches, and impaired mobility. It should be considered a marker for potentially lethal trauma because it is associated with an 11% mortality rate from associated injuries [73–75].

The Anderson and Montesano system is used to classify occipital condyle fractures [76] (see **Figure 14**).

Treatment includes cervical orthosis for type 1, type 2, and stable type 3 fractures [75].

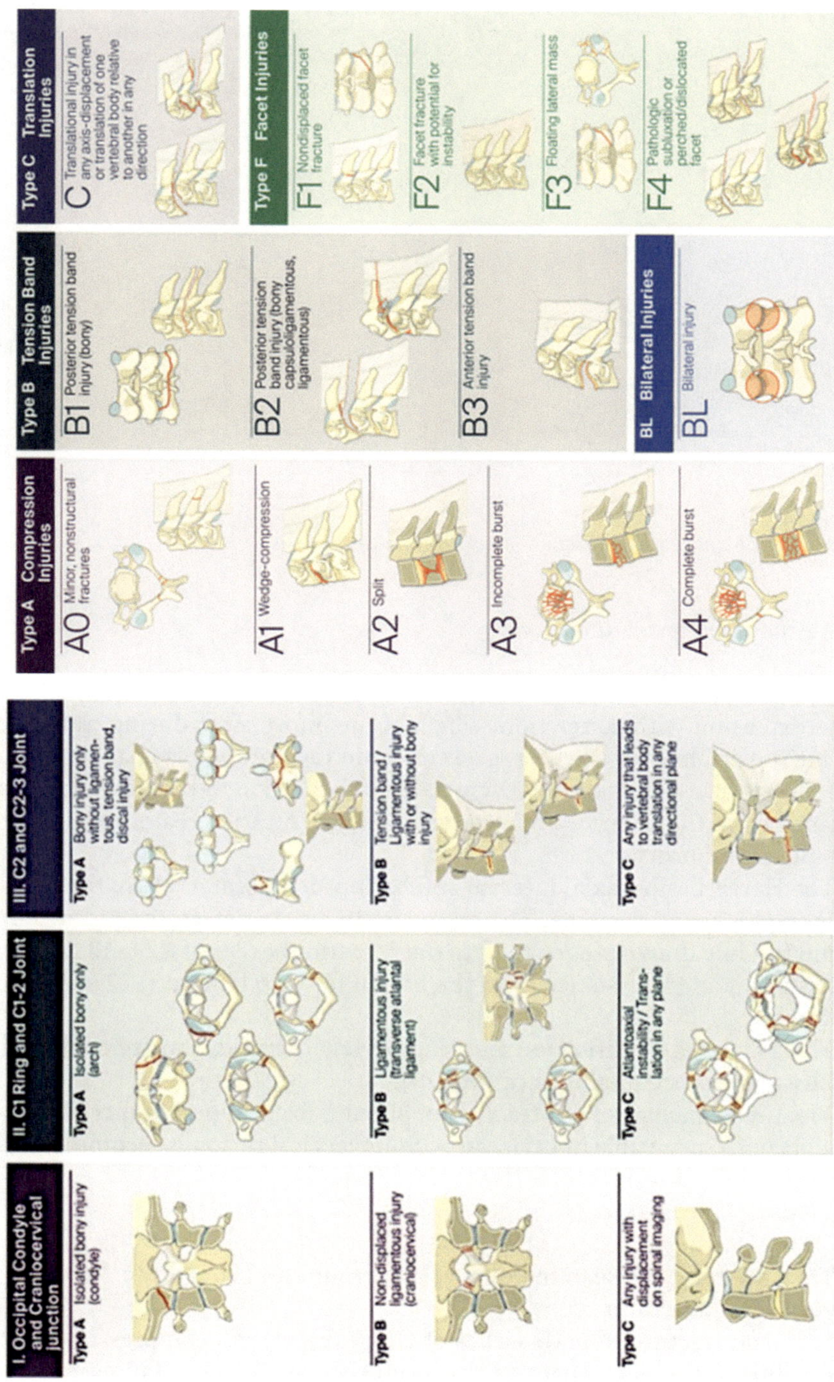

Figure 13.
AO Spine Classification System (reproduced with permission from https://www.aofoundation.org/).

	Type I	Type II	Type III
Description	**Comminuted fracture** +/- minimal displacement of fragments.	**Linear skull fracture** that extends to involve the occipital condyle.	**Avulsion fracture** of the condyle near the alar ligament.
Mechanism	Axial loading-impacted fracture.	Direct blow.	Rotation and/or contralateral bending.
Stability	**STABLE**, unless, bilateral	**STABLE**	**POTENTIALLY UNSTABLE**

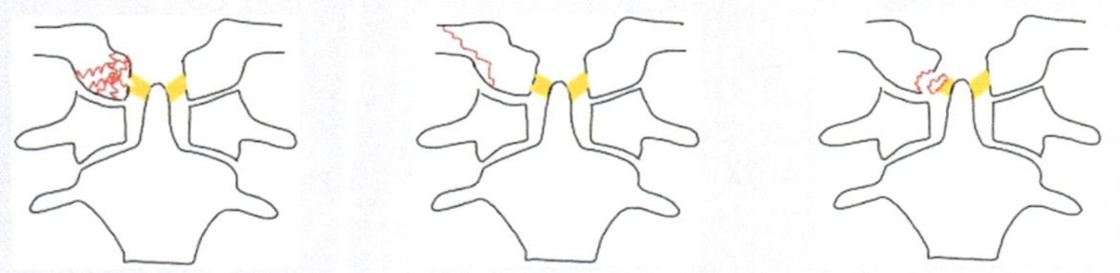

Figure 14.
Anderson and Montesano classification of occipital condyle fractures.

5.1.2 Atlanto-occipital dislocation

A highly unstable injury, the most common mechanism of injury is hyperextension with distraction, which occurs most often during traffic accidents. It's incompatible with life. Diagnosis on plain radiography is challenging [77, 78].

Powers ratio – divides the distance from the basion to the posterior arch by the distance from the anterior arch to the opisthion. A ratio greater than 1 suggests possible anterior dislocation.

The Harris basion-axial interval and basion-dental interval are the most sensitive radiographic measurements. They measure two parameters: the distance from the basion to a line drawn tangentially to the posterior border of C2 (>12 mm or <4 mm is abnormal), and the distance from the basion to the odontoid (>12 mm is considered abnormal).

The Traynelis classification and Harborview classification are commonly used to classify atlanto-occipital dislocation [79].

Treatment includes light traction of about 5 lbs in type 1 and type 3 injuries. In patients with survivable injuries, an occipitocervical fusion is recommended [77, 78].

5.1.3 Atlas (C1) fractures

They are typically seen in younger age groups and constitute 2% to 13% of cervical spine fractures.

Jefferson fracture of both arches of C1 (*Jefferson*) is a compression fracture that occurs during a direct impact on the head, such as diving or falling from a height. This injury does not cause a neurological outburst because the C1 ring is very wide. The fracture is unstable, and surgical treatment or halo immobilization is indicated [80, 81] (see **Figure 15**).

DOI: http://dx.doi.org/10.5772/intechopen.1014132

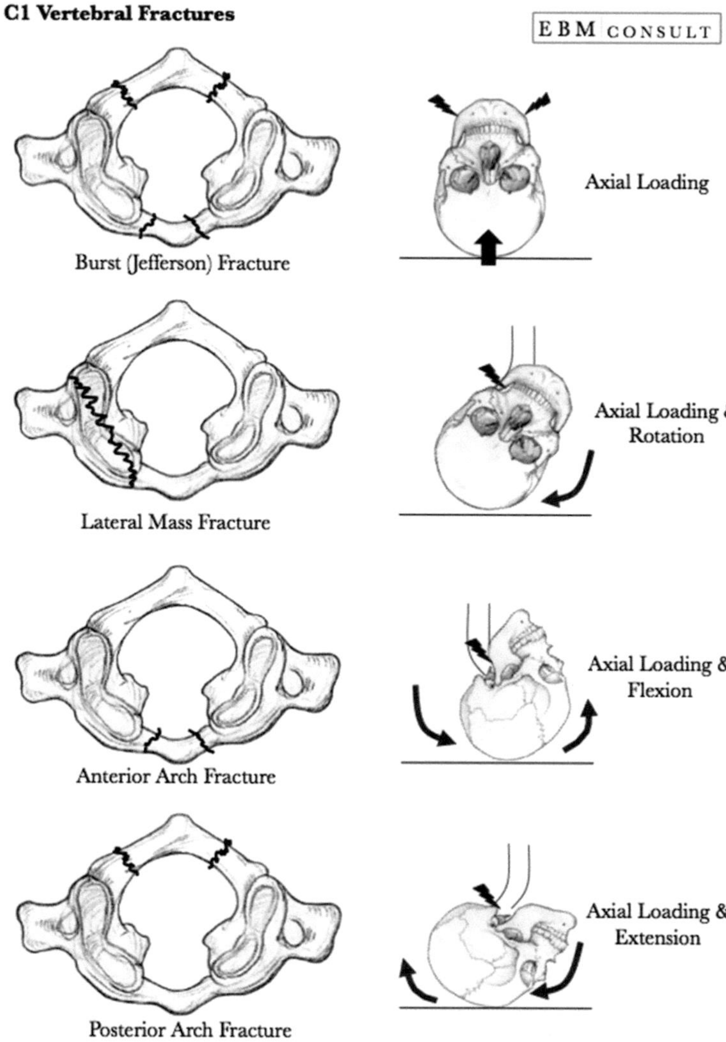

Figure 15.
Fracture of the C1 vertebra (reproduced with permission from https://www.ebmconsult.com).

Treatment for isolated anterior or posterior arch fractures, lateral mass fractures, and transverse process fractures can be nonsurgical – using a cervical collar for 6 to 12 weeks. This approach is also applicable in burst fractures involving both anterior and posterior arches with an intact transverse ligament (less than 7 mm of combined lateral overhang of lateral masses). Treatment for unstable injuries (combined lateral mass displacement greater than 7 mm) includes bed rest with traction; additionally, surgical treatment has become widely accepted [81].

5.1.4 Odontoid fractures

A frequent fracture, which is caused by the mechanism of hyperflexion, occurs when falling on the head or in a traffic accident. In people over 70 years of age, these

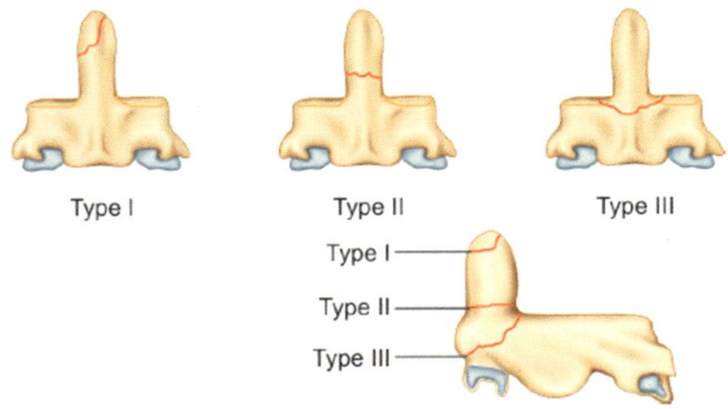

Figure 16.
Anderson and D'Alonzo classification of the C2 fracture from modern Techniques in Spine Surgery, Chapter 14: Technique of Odontoid Screw Fixation for type 2 Odontoid Fractures; DOI: 10.5005/jp/books/1,2509_15.

are the most common fractures of the cervical spine. They result in neurological failure in more than 50% of cases [82, 83].

The Anderson and d'Alonzo classification is used for odontoid fractures, and the Roy-Camille classification [82] **(Figure 16)**.

Treatment is conservative for type 1 and type 3 – cervical collar for 6 to 12 weeks, or operative in type 2, depending on fracture characteristics and the patient population. The high nonunion rate – 32% – and the poor tolerance of halo vests by elderly patients mean these patients should be considered for early C1–C2 fusion [83].

5.1.5 Traumatic spondylolisthesis of the axis ("hangman's fracture")

The most common fracture of the upper cervical spine occurs due to hyperextension of the neck, whereby, due to a bilateral fracture of the pars interarticularis of C2, the vertebral body of C2 slips in relation to the vertebral body of C3. It is most often caused by traffic accidents, injuries in contact sports, or when jumping on the head (diving). There is usually no neurological outburst, or it is minimal [84, 85].

Modified Effendi classification by Levine and Edwards is used [86] (see **Figure 17**).

Treatment is surgical in type 2 fractures with severe angulation and type 3 fractures with disruption of the C2–C3 disk and/or facet dislocation. Surgical options include anterior C2–C3 fusion, posterior C1–C3 fusion, and bilateral C2 pars interarticularis screws [84, 85].

5.1.6 Fractures of the subaxial spine (C3–C7)

There are several classifications of injuries to the subaxial cervical spine. The simplest division of injuries is into fractures (here the simpler – compressive – and more complex – explosive "burst" fractures are distinguished) and dislocations (which can be unilateral, if there is a slip of up to 25% of the length of the vertebral body, and bilateral, if it is a slip over 25% of the length of the vertebral body) [87].

The Allen–Ferguson Classification is one of the generally accepted classifications, which divides all injuries of the subaxial cervical spine into six

Classification	Definition	Mechanism
Effendi		
Type I	Isolated hairline fracture of ring of axis	Axial loading and hyperextension
Type II	Displacement of anterior fragment and abnormal disk below axis	Further hyperextension and rebound flexion
Type III	Displacement of anterior fragment andlocked facet at C2–C3	Flexion and rebound extension
Levine and Edwards		
Type I	Non displaced fracture (<3 mm)	Hyperextension and axial loading
Type II	Significant angulation (>11 degrees) and translation (>3 mm)	Hyperextension, axial loading and rebound flexion
Type IIa	Very severe angulation without translation	Flexion-distraction

Figure 17.
Modified Effendi classification by Levine and Edwards A study on management of Hangman's fracture – scientific figure on ResearchGate. Available from: https://www.researchgate.net/figure/classification-of-hangmans-fracture_tbl1_331792182 [accessed 9 Sept 2025]

types: compression-flexion, vertical compression, distraction-flexion, compression-extension, distraction-extension, and lateral-flexion [88].

The most recent classification is the Subaxial Injury Classification and Severity Scale (SLICS). This classification takes into account three factors: the morphology of the fracture (0–4 points), the integrity of the disko-ligamentous complex (0–2 points), and the neurological status of the injured person (0–4 points). If the number of points is greater than 5, then surgical treatment is indicated [89].

(1) A compressive "wedge" fracture of the subaxial cervical spine is caused by the action of a moderate axial force. Then, there is a lowering of the front part of the vertebral body. The posterior elements are intact, and spinal cord injuries are rare, so therapy is conservative – immobilization for 6 to 12 weeks.

(2) An explosive "burst" fracture is caused by the action of an axial force of very high intensity, whereby an "explosion" of the vertebral body occurs. Bone fragments move in all directions, and, due to damage to the posterior longitudinal ligament, the spinal cord is compressed, and neurological failure occurs. In this case, the treatment is operative.

(3) Teardrop fracture is a flexion axial load injury characterized by a fracture of the anterior-inferior portion of a vertebra as it is driven caudally and into flexion, causing retropulsion of the remaining vertebral body into the spinal canal.

(4) Facet fracture-dislocation of the subaxial cervical spine involves the loss of contact between the articular surfaces. It can be unilateral if there is a slip of up to 25% of the length of the vertebral body, or bilateral if the slip is greater than 25%. The injury is unstable, especially in the flexion position, so surgery is indicated. Due to the instability and high risk of spinal cord injury, it is necessary to provide initial treatment for such an injury, which is skeletal traction.

(5) Fracture of the spinous process of C7 (*Clay-shoveler* fracture) can be caused by a direct force in the region of the spinous process, or indirectly by a strong contraction of the paravertebral musculature. It's mostly an isolated injury. It is not accompanied by spinal cord injuries. Therapy is conservative.

6. Thoracolumbar fractures

6.1 Classification of injuries of the thoracolumbar spine

The first serious classification is the one based on the concept of three pillars: the anterior pillar (involving the anterior half of the vertebral body), the middle pillar (involving the posterior half of the vertebral body and the spinal canal), and the posterior pillar (involving the laminae, pedicles, facet joints, transverse and spinal processes). A combination of injuries to either two pillars is considered an unstable injury, where surgical treatment is indicated.

In practice, the following classification is the most popular:

(1) Compressive fracture – The lower lumbar region has a greater ability to tolerate flexion moments, so anterior column failure should raise the suspicion of posterior ligamentous injury, especially when more than 50% loss of vertebral height is seen.

(2) Explosive "burst" fracture – are more common than compressive fractures, and most injuries occur with the spine in a neutral position, resulting in axial loading of the anterior and middle columns. The incidence of neurological deficit is much lower in the lower lumbar spine because the spinal cord ends above this level, and the cauda equina and nerve roots are more tolerant of compression.

(3) "Chance" fracture – represents a horizontal avulsion fracture. It is an unstable spinal injury, most often at the thoracolumbar junction (T12–L2), caused by a rapid flexion-distraction mechanism, such as in a car accident with a lap belt. It is a horizontal fracture through the posterior elements (spinous process, pedicles) and the vertebral body, often involving ligaments as well.

(4) Flexion –distraction injuries – For the lumbar spine, these fractures are most common at L2 and L4.

(5) Translational injuries (luxation fractures)

It is worth mentioning another classification that has found application in clinical practice, and that is the Thoracolumbar Injury Classification System (TLICS). This classification takes into account three factors: the morphology of the fracture (0–4 points), the integrity of the disko-ligamentous complex (0–2 points), and the neurological status of the injured person (0–4 points). If the number of points is greater than 5, then surgical treatment is indicated [90].

The AO Classification System has largely replaced the TLICS and Denis classification scale [91, 92]. **Figure 18.**

6.2 Treatment of thoracolumbar fractures

Treatment for patients who are neurologically intact, who have less than 25 degrees of kyphosis, less than 50% loss of vertebral height, and less than 50% canal compromise, and who have an intact posterior ligamentous complex is nonsurgical – orthosis for three months.

Surgical treatment is indicated for unstable fractures and/or patients with neurological deficits. Patients with unstable burst fractures, including failure of the posterior ligamentous complex, fracture-dislocation, and fractures with significant rotational displacement, should undergo initial posterior stabilization [42, 43, 45].

7. Sacral fractures

Due to its unique anatomical location, injuries to the sacrum may result in deformity, neurologic deficit, and altered neurological function of the bowel/bladder and lower extremities.

Initial evaluation of high-energy suspected sacral fractures involves log-rolling during the secondary survey, with inspection and palpation of the spinal column up

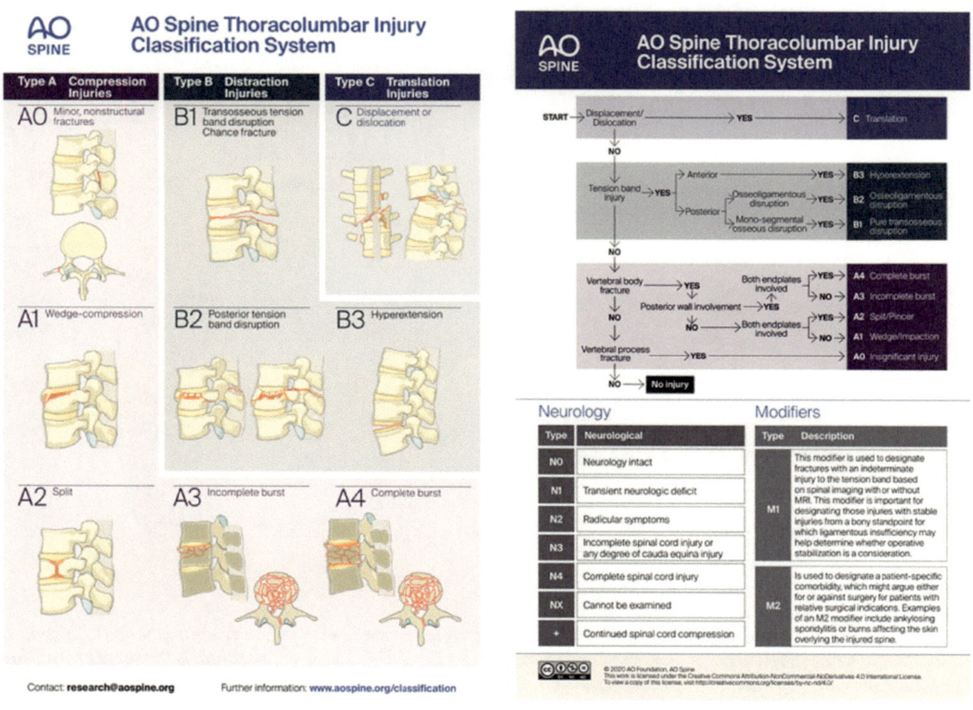

Figure 18.
AO Spine Classification System (reproduced with permission from https://www.aofoundation.org/).

to the coccyx. Additionally, neurological examination of the lower extremities and bowel/bladder function is required. Sacral fractures are often associated with root deficits [93].

The Denis classification, or AO Sacral Injury Classification System, is used for sacral fractures [94, 95]; see **Figure 19** and **Figure 20**.

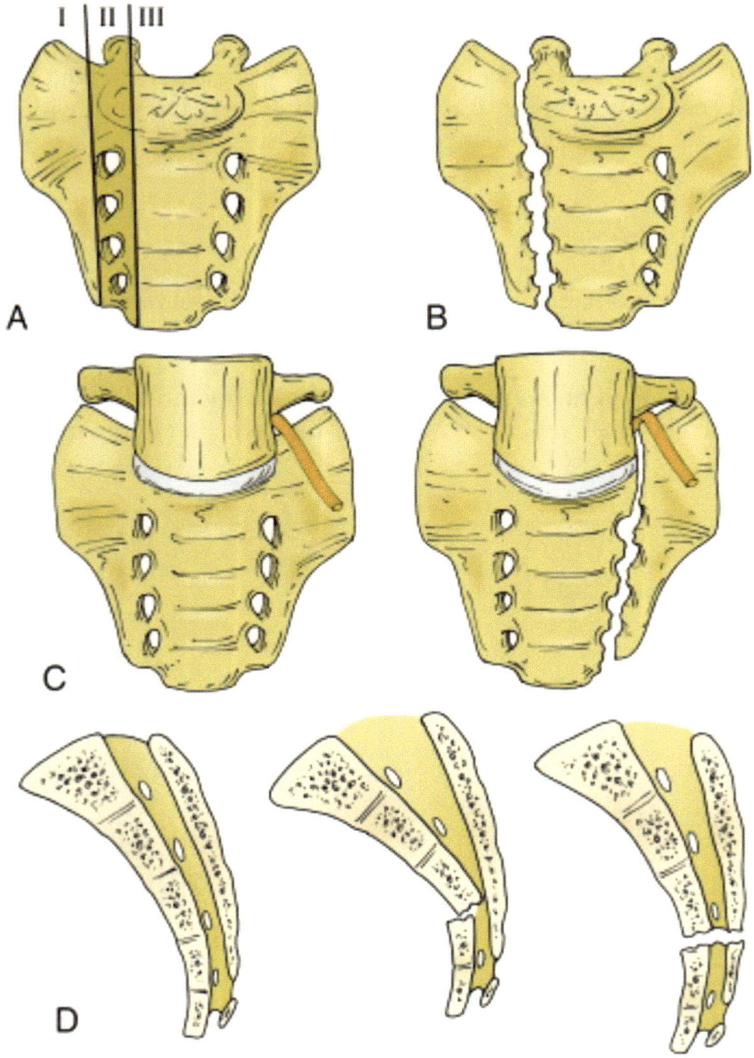

Figure 19.
The Denis classification of sacral fractures. (a) The three zones (zone I, alar region fracture; zone II, foraminal region fracture; zone III, central canal region fracture). (b) Zone II fracture going through the sacral foramina. (c) Image showing normal sacral anatomy with reference to the L-5 nerve root (left) and a zone II fracture causing compression of the L-5 nerve root (right). (d) Sagittal views of normal sacrum (left), a zone III burst fracture (middle), and a zone III fracture dislocation (right). Reproduced with permission from Denis F., Davis S., Comfort T. Sacral fractures: An important problem: Retrospective analysis of 236 cases. Clin Orthop Relat Res 227:67–81, 1988.

DOI: http://dx.doi.org/10.5772/intechopen.1014132

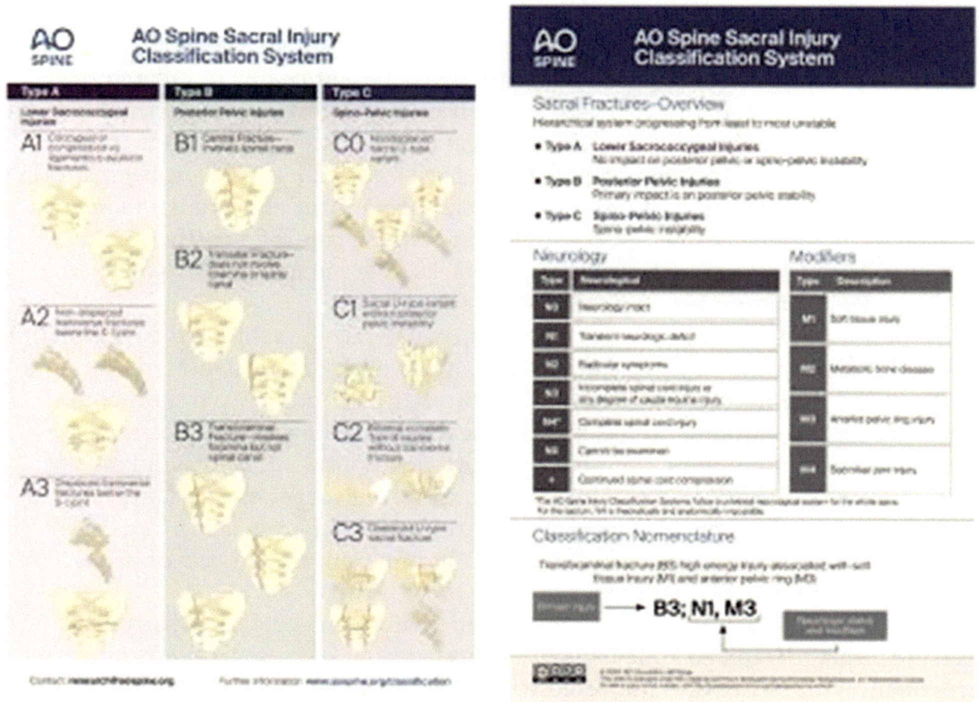

Figure 20.
AO Spine Classification System (reproduced with permission from https://www.aofoundation.org/).

7.1 Treatment of sacral fractures

Treatment depends on the location and pattern of the fracture, the presence of impaction, the integrity of the L5–S1 facet, associated pelvic fractures, and neurologic deficit.

Treatment of Zone 1 and Zone 2 displaced fractures is followed by percutaneous iliosacral screw fixation; however, in Zone 2, to avoid further injury to the sacral root, the iliosacral screw should not be placed in compression.

Zone 3 injuries commonly involve open-book pelvic fracture patterns with diastasis anteriorly and gapping at the sacral fracture posteriorly. Initial treatment should address the anterior pelvic ring disruption, followed by posterior screw fixation if necessary.

Indications for spinopelvic fixation include the presence of vertical shear or disruption of the L5–S1 facets.

8. Postoperative care and rehabilitation

Early rehabilitation is crucial to preventing thromboembolic and other complications, especially in patients with neurological deficits.

When it comes to patients who have an injury that is treated non-operatively and do not have a neurological deficit, early rehabilitation treatment is started immediately after obtaining adequate immobilization. When it comes to minor injuries such as fractures of the transverse processes and spinous processes (according to the AO classification, they are AOA0), after six weeks, the immobilization is removed, and rehabilitation treatment begins in inpatient conditions or on an outpatient basis. When it comes to vertebral body fractures that are treated non-operatively, and neurological findings are normal, after three months, the immobilization is removed, and rehabilitation treatment begins. While wearing immobilization, it is advised to avoid lifting loads and sudden movements, as well as prolonged sitting and standing due to the heavy load on the spinal column. At the regular controls after two weeks, one month, and six weeks, the healing of the fracture is monitored by X-ray.

When it comes to patients treated operatively, early rehabilitation treatment is started either on the same day of surgery or the next day in the ward. Patients undergoing minimally invasive surgery (lumbar diskectomy, percutaneous vertebroplasty, vertebra biopsy) are verticalized on the same day of the intervention and go home the next day with behavioral advice (avoidance of heavy lifting and sudden movements). Considering that these patients have an operative wound, after removing the sutures, usually two weeks after the operation, rehabilitation treatment begins in inpatient conditions or as an ambulatory type.

A special challenge is presented by patients with neurological impairment (quadriplegia, paraplegia, quadriparesis, paraparesis). In these patients, operative treatment is almost always indicated within 24 to 48 hours of the injury, and immediately after the operative treatment, they are included in early intensive rehabilitation treatment both in the ward and then in institutions that specialize in these conditions. This includes intensive physical therapy, exercises, and prevention of decubitus. Regular follow-ups include checks 2 weeks after discharge, 1 month, 6 months, and 12 months [96–98].

9. Conclusion

Spinal trauma, with associated injuries to other organs and with spinal cord injury, presents a great challenge for both diagnosis and treatment. It is crucial to recognize spinal injury in a polytraumatized patient, as well as to diagnose it in a timely manner.

Take-home messages are: Patients with ankylosing spondylitis have an increased risk of spinal fractures as a result of minor trauma; Brown-Séquard syndrome has the best prognosis after SCI; Abdominal visceral injuries occur in 50% of patients with flexion-distraction injuries in the thoracolumbar spine; Early decompression significantly improves ASIA score; In patients with SCI, hypotension should be avoided, and mean arterial blood pressure should be maintained at 85 to 90 mm Hg to prevent secondary SCI; Most lower lumbar spine fractures can be treated nonsurgically.

Conflict of Interest

The author declares no conflict of interest.

DOI: http://dx.doi.org/10.5772/intechopen.1014132

Author details

Slavisa Zagorac[1,2]

1 Faculty of Medicine, University of Belgrade, Belgrade, Serbia

2 Clinic for Orthopedic Surgery and Traumatology, University Clinical Center of Serbia, Belgrade, Serbia

*Address all correspondence to: slavisa.zagorac@gmail.com

References

[1] Cramer GD, Darby SA. Clinical Anatomy of the Spine, Spinal Cord, and ANS. 3rd ed. St. Louis, Missouri: Mosby; 2017

[2] Gardner E, Gray DJ, O'Rahhily R. Anatomy. Philadelphia: WB Saunders; 1975

[3] Woon JT, Stringer MD. Clinical anatomy of the coccyx: A systematic review. Clinical Anatomy. 2012;**25**(2):158–167. DOI: 10.1002/ca.21216

[4] Bican O, Minagar A, Pruitt AA. The spinal cord: A review of functional neuroanatomy. Neurologic Clinics. 2013;**31**(1):1–18. DOI: 10.1016/j.ncl.2012.09.009

[5] Santillan A, Nacarino V, Greenberg E, Riina HA, Gobin YP, Patsalides A. Vascular anatomy of the spinal cord. Journal of NeuroInterventional Surgery. 2012;**4**(1):67–74. DOI: 10.1136/neurintsurg-2011-010018

[6] Bogduk N. Functional anatomy of the spine. Handbook of Clinical Neurology. 2016;**136**:675–688. DOI: 10.1016/B978-0-444-53486-6.00032-6

[7] Goris BC, Kuipers M, De Vries J, Wever DJ, Verkerke GJ, Veldhuizen AG. On the determination of the angular orientation of a vertebra. Journal of Biomechanical Engineering. 2002;**124**(1):134–136. DOI: 10.1115/1.1431265

[8] Bonczar M, Koszewski J, Czarnota W, Dziedzic M, Ostrowski P, Możdżeń K, Murawska A, Hajdyła P, Walocha A, Walocha E, Walocha J, Koziej M. The morphology of the lumbar vertebrae: A systematic review with meta-analysis of 1481 individuals with implications for spine surgery. Surgical and Radiologic Anatomy. 2024;**47**(1):22. DOI: 10.1007/s00276-024-03509-4

[9] Izzo R, Guarnieri G, Guglielmi G, Muto M. Biomechanics of the spine. Part I: Spinal stability. European Journal of Radiology. 2013;**82**(1):118–126. DOI: 10.1016/j.ejrad.2012.07.024

[10] Oxland TR. Fundamental biomechanics of the spine–What we have learned in the past 25 years and future directions. Journal of Biomechanics. 2016;**49**(6):817–832. DOI: 10.1016/j.jbiomech.2015.10.035

[11] Bland JH, Boushey DR. Anatomy and physiology of the cervical spine. Seminars in Arthritis and Rheumatism. 1990;**20**(1):1–20. DOI: 10.1016/0049-0172(90)90090-3

[12] Resnick DK, Weller SJ, Benzel EC. Biomechanics of the thoracolumbar spine. Neurosurgery Clinics of North America. 1997;**8**(4):455–469

[13] Byrd SE, Comiskey EM. Postnatal maturation and radiology of the growing spine. Neurosurgery Clinics of North America. 2007;**18**(3):431–461. DOI: 10.1016/j.nec.2007.05.002

[14] Kumar R, Lim J, Mekary RA, Rattani A, Dewan MC, Sharif SY, Osorio-Fonseca E, Park KB. Traumatic spinal injury: Global epidemiology and worldwide volume. World Neurosurgery. 2018;**113**:e345–e363. DOI: 10.1016/j.wneu.2018.02.033

[15] J DPM. Epidemiology of osteoporotic fractures: Vertebral and

non-vertebral fractures. Rev Osteoporos Metab Miner. 2010;**2**(5):8–12

[16] Tran NT, Watson NA, Tencer AF, Ching RP, Anderson PA. Mechanism of the burst fracture in the thoracolumbar spine. The effect of loading rate. Spine (Philadelphia, Pennsylvania 1976). 1995;**20**(18):1984–1988. DOI: 10.1097/00007632-199509150-00004

[17] Kumar S, Kumar P, Patralekh MK, Srinivasan R, Agarwal A, Boruah T. Fracture-dislocation of the thoracolumbar spine without neurological deficit: A report of two cases and literature review. Spinal Cord Series and Cases. 2020;**6**(1):67. DOI: 10.1038/s41394-020-0315-4

[18] Dowdell J, Kim J, Overley S, Hecht A. Biomechanics and common mechanisms of injury of the cervical spine. Handbook of Clinical Neurology. 2018;**158**:337–344. DOI: 10.1016/B978-0-444-63954-7.00031-8

[19] Smith D, Bowden T. Using the ABCDE approach to assess the deteriorating patient. Nursing Standard. 2017;**32**(14):51–63. DOI: 10.7748/ns.2017.e11030

[20] Lodier F. ABCDE, une nouvelle approche de prise en charge aux urgences [ABCDE, a new approach to patient management in emergency departments]. Soins. 2018;**63**(825):27–29. DOI: 10.1016/j.soin.2018.03.006

[21] Moraes FDS, Marengo LL, Moura MDG, Bergamaschi CC, de Sá Del Fiol F, Lopes LC, Silva MT, Barberato-Filho S. ABCDE and ABCDEF care bundles: A systematic review of the implementation process in intensive care units. Medicine (Baltimore). 2022;**101**(25):e29499. DOI: 10.1097/MD.0000000000029499

[22] Connor D, Greaves I, Porter K, Bloch M. consensus group, Faculty of Pre-Hospital Care. Pre-hospital spinal immobilisation: An initial consensus statement. Emergency Medicine Journal. 2013;**30**(12):1067–1069. DOI: 10.1136/emermed-2013-203207

[23] Hood N, Considine J. Spinal immobilisaton in pre-hospital and emergency care: A systematic review of the literature. Australasian Emergency Nursing Journal. 2015;**18**(3):118–137. DOI: 10.1016/j.aenj.2015.03.003

[24] Kwan I, Bunn F, Roberts I. Spinal immobilisation for trauma patients. The Cochrane Database of Systematic Reviews. 2001;**2001**(2):CD002803. DOI: 10.1002/14651858.CD002803

[25] Oosterwold JT, Sagel DC, van Grunsven PM, Holla M, de Man-van Ginkel J, Berben S. The characteristics and pre-hospital management of blunt trauma patients with suspected spinal column injuries: A retrospective observational study. European Journal of Trauma and Emergency Surgery. 2017;**43**(4):513–524. DOI: 10.1007/s00068-016-0688-z

[26] Pandor A, Essat M, Sutton A, Fuller G, Reid S, Smith JE, Fothergill R, Surendra Kumar D, Kolias A, Hutchinson P, Perkins GD, Wilson MH, Lecky F. Cervical spine immobilisation following blunt trauma in pre-hospital and emergency care: A systematic review. PLoS One. 2024;**19**(4):e0302127. DOI: 10.1371/journal.pone.0302127

[27] Wiles MD, Iliff HA, Brooks K, Da Silva EJ, Donnellon M, Gardner A, Harris M, Leech C, Mathieu S, Moor P, Prisco L, Rivett K, Tait F, El-Boghdadly K. Airway management in patients with suspected or confirmed cervical spine

injury: Guidelines from the Difficult Airway Society (DAS. Association of Anaesthetists (Aoa), British Society of Orthopaedic Anaesthetists (BSOA), Intensive Care Society (ICS), Neuro Anaesthesia and Critical Care Society (NACCS), Faculty of Prehospital Care and Royal College of Emergency Medicine (RCEM). Anaesthesia. 2024;**79**(8):856–868. DOI: 10.1111/anae.16290

[28] Vickery D. The use of the spinal board after the pre-hospital phase of trauma management. Emergency Medicine Journal. 2001;**18**(1):51–54. DOI: 10.1136/emj.18.1.51

[29] Purvis TA, Carlin B, Driscoll P. The definite risks and questionable benefits of liberal pre-hospital spinal immobilisation. The American Journal of Emergency Medicine. 2017;**35**(6):860–866. DOI: 10.1016/j.ajem.2017.01.045

[30] Ahn H, Singh J, Nathens A, MacDonald RD, Travers A, Tallon J, Fehlings MG, Yee A. Pre-hospital care management of a potential spinal cord injured patient: A systematic review of the literature and evidence-based guidelines. Journal of Neurotrauma. 2011;**28**(8):1341–1361. DOI: 10.1089/neu.2009.1168

[31] Nilhas A, Helmer SD, Drake RM, Reyes J, Morriss M, Haan JM. Pre-hospital spinal immobilization: Neurological outcomes for spinal motion restriction versus spinal immobilization. Kansas Journal of Medicine. 2022;**15**(1):119–122. DOI: 10.17161/kjm.vol15.16213

[32] Khan SA, Khalid S, Khan AA, Javed Z, Hussain J, Khan Afridi EA, Haroon MZ, Aurangzeb A. Level of pre-tertiary care hospital management of traumatic spinal cord injured patients; where do we stand? Journal of Ayub Medical College, Abbottabad: JAMC. 2021;**33**(2):305–310

[33] Hess T, Hirschfeld S, Thietje R, Lönnecker S, Kerner T, Stuhr M. Die akute traumatische Querschnittslähmung - Wie ist präklinisch vorzugehen? [Pre-hospital care management of acute spinal cord injury]. AINS - Anästhesiologie Intensivmedizin Notfallmedizin Schmerztherapie. 2016;**51**(4):226–237. DOI: 10.1055/s-0042-105016

[34] American Spinal Injury Association (ASIA) Impairment Scale. Physiopedia. 2025, June 15. Available from: https://www.physio-pedia.com/index.php?title=American_Spinal_Injury_Association_(ASIA)_Impairment_Scale&oldid=369724 [Accessed: 2025-October-26]

[35] Baratloo A, Ahmadzadeh K, Forouzanfar MM, Yousefifard M, Farhang RM, Hashemi B, Aghili SH. NEXUS vs. Canadian C-spine rule (CCR) in predicting cervical spine injuries; A systematic review and meta-analysis. Archives of Academic Emergency Medicine. 2023;**11**(1):e66. DOI: 10.22037/aaem.v11i1.2143

[36] Saragiotto BT, Maher CG, Lin CWC, Verhagen AP, Goergen S, Michaleff ZA. Canadian C-spine rule and the National Emergency X-Radiography Utilization Study (NEXUS) for detecting clinically important cervical spine injury following blunt trauma. Cochrane Database of Systematic Reviews. 2018;**2018**(4):CD012989. DOI: 10.1002/14651858.CD012989

[37] Schnadthorst PG, Lankes C, Schulze C. Konservative Behandlung

traumatisch bedingter Frakturen der Halswirbelsäule mit Orthesen – Ein Review [Conservative treatment of trauma-associated fractures of the cervical spine with orthoses-A review]. Die Unfallchirurgie. 2023;**126**(12):943–950. DOI: 10.1007/s00113-022-01261-1

[38] Delcourt T, Bégué T, Saintyves G, Mebtouche N, Cottin P. Management of upper cervical spine fractures in elderly patients: Current trends and outcomes. Injury. 2015;**46**(Suppl 1):S24–7. DOI: 10.1016/S0020-1383(15)70007-0

[39] Bhushan A, Beland A, Poelstra C, Butterfield J, Angel M, Cheung T, Plater E, Guha D, Pahuta M, Macedo LG. Immobilization protocols for the treatment of cervical spine fracture: A scoping review. The Spine Journal. 2024;**24**(9):1571–1594. DOI: 10.1016/j.spinee.2024.05.012

[40] Uche EO, Nwankwo OE, Okorie E, Muobike A. Skull traction for cervical spinal injury in Enugu: A 5-year retrospective multicenter analysis of the clinical outcomes of patients treated with two common devices. Nigerian Journal of Clinical Practice. 2016;**19**(5):580–584. DOI: 10.4103/1119-3077.188713

[41] Parney IF, Allen PB, Petruk KC, Howard H. Hepburn and the development of skull tongs for cervical spine traction. Neurosurgery. 2000;**47**(6):1430–1433

[42] Wood KB, Buttermann GR, Phukan R, Harrod CC, Mehbod A, Shannon B, Bono CM, Harris MB. Operative compared with nonoperative treatment of a thoracolumbar burst fracture without neurological deficit: A prospective randomized study with follow-up at sixteen to twenty-two years. Journal of Bone and Joint Surgery. 2015;**97**(1):3–9. DOI: 10.2106/JBJS.N.00226

[43] Wood KB, Li W, Lebl DR, Ploumis A. Management of thoracolumbar spine fractures. The Spine Journal. 2014;**14**(1):145–164. DOI: 10.1016/j.spinee.2012.10.041

[44] Joaquim AF, Patel AA, Schroeder GD, Vaccaro AR. A simplified treatment algorithm for treating thoracic and lumbar spine trauma. The Journal of Spinal Cord Medicine. 2019;**42**(4):416–422. DOI: 10.1080/10790268.2018.1433267

[45] Rampersaud YR, Annand N, Dekutoski MB. Use of minimally invasive surgical techniques in the management of thoracolumbar trauma: Current concepts. Spine (Philadelphia, Pennsylvania 1976). 2006;**31**(11 Suppl):S96–102. DOI: 10.1097/01.brs.0000218250.51148.5b

[46] Koreckij T, Park DK, Fischgrund J. Minimally invasive spine surgery in the treatment of thoracolumbar and lumbar spine trauma. Neurosurgical Focus. 2014;**37**(1):E11. DOI: 10.3171/2014.5.FOCUS1494

[47] Filippiadis DK, Marcia S, Masala S, Deschamps F, Kelekis A. Percutaneous vertebroplasty and kyphoplasty: Current status, new developments and old controversies. CardioVascular and Interventional Radiology. 2017;**40**(12):1815–1823. DOI: 10.1007/s00270-017-1779-x

[48] Peh WC, Munk PL, Rashid F, Gilula LA. Percutaneous vertebral augmentation: Vertebroplasty, kyphoplasty and skyphoplasty. Radiologic Clinics of North America. 2008;**46**(3):611–35,vii. DOI: 10.1016/j.rcl.2008.05.005

[49] Hoppenfeld S, de Boer P, Buckley R. Surgical Exposures in Orthopaedics: The Anatomic Approach. 5e Lippincott Williams & Wilkins, a Wolters Kluwer Bu; 2016. Available from: https://orthopaedics.lwwhealthlibrary.com/book.aspx?bookid=1935§ionid=0 [Accessed: 2025-October-26]

[50] Arumalla K, Bansal H, Jadeja J, Batish A, Deora H, Tripathi M, Mohindra S, Behari S. Anterior approach to the cervical spine: Elegance lies in its simplicity. Asian Journal of Neurosurgery. 2021;**16**(4):669–684. DOI: 10.4103/ajns.AJNS_313_20

[51] Razi A, Saleh H, DeLacure MD, Kim Y. Anterior approach to the subaxial cervical spine: Pearls and pitfalls. Journal of the American Academy of Orthopaedic Surgeons. 2021;**29**(5):189–195. DOI: 10.5435/JAAOS-D-17-00891

[52] Liu JK, Das K. Posterior fusion of the subaxial cervical spine: Indications and techniques. Neurosurgical Focus. 2001;**10**(4):E7. DOI: 10.3171/foc.2001.10.4.8

[53] Haupt S, Cornaz F, Falkowski AL, Widmer J, Farshad M. Biomechanical considerations of the posterior surgical approach to the lumbar spine. The Spine Journal. 2022;**22**(12):2066–2071. DOI: 10.1016/j.spinee.2022.08.006

[54] Zhu Q, Shi F, Cai W, Bai J, Fan J, Yang H. Comparison of anterior versus posterior approach in the treatment of thoracolumbar fractures: A systematic review. International Surgery. 2015;**100**(6):1124–1133. DOI: 10.9738/INTSURG-D-14-00135.1

[55] Tan T, Huang MS, Mathew J, Fitzgerald M, Chan P, Hunn MK, Tee J. Anterior versus posterior approach in the management of AO Type B1 & B2 traumatic thoracolumbar fractures: A level 1 trauma centre study. Journal of Clinical Neuroscience. 2020;**72**:219–223. DOI: 10.1016/j.jocn.2019.11.039

[56] Chen ZW, Ding ZQ, Zhai WL, Lian KJ, Kang LQ, Guo LX, Liu H, Lin B. Anterior versus posterior approach in the treatment of chronic thoracolumbar fractures. Orthopedics. 2012;**35**(2):e219–24. DOI: 10.3928/01477447-20120123-05

[57] Schoenen J. Clinical anatomy of the spinal cord. Neurologic Clinics. 1991;**9**(3):503–532

[58] Pearce JM. The development of spinal cord anatomy. European Neurology. 2008;**59**(6):286–291. DOI: 10.1159/000121417

[59] Kunam VK, Velayudhan V, Chaudhry ZA, Bobinski M, Smoker WRK, Reede DL. Incomplete cord syndromes: Clinical and imaging review. Radiographics. 2018;**38**(4):1201–1222. DOI: 10.1148/rg.2018170178

[60] Carr MT, Harrop JS, Houten JK. Traumatic Central Cord Syndrome. Clinical Spine Surgery. 2024;**37**(9):379–387. DOI: 10.1097/BSD.0000000000001703

[61] Avila MJ, Hurlbert RJ. Central cord syndrome redefined. Neurosurgery Clinics of North America. 2021;**32**(3):353–363. DOI: 10.1016/j.nec.2021.03.007

[62] Pearl NA, Weisbrod LJ, Dubensky L. Anterior Cord Syndrome (Archived). In: StatPearls. Treasure Island (FL): StatPearls Publishing; 2025

[63] Khan MM, Munakomi S, Dalal K. Ventral Cord Syndrome. In: StatPearls. Treasure Island (FL): StatPearls Publishing; 2025. Available from: https://www.ncbi.nlm.nih.gov/books/NBK541011/ [Accessed: 2025-November-7]

[64] Shams S, Davidson CL, Arain A. Brown-Séquard Syndrome. In: StatPearls. Treasure Island (FL): StatPearls Publishing; 2024. Available from: https://www.ncbi.nlm.nih.gov/books/NBK538135/ [Accessed: 2024-Febuary-27]

[65] Franges EZ. Solving the puzzle of Brown-Séquard syndrome. Nursing. 2021;**51**(4):62–66. DOI: 10.1097/01.NURSE.0000733960.67995.78

[66] McKinley W, Hills A, Sima A. Posterior cord syndrome: Demographics and rehabilitation outcomes. The Journal of Spinal Cord Medicine. 2021;**44**(2):241–246. DOI: 10.1080/10790268.2019.1585135

[67] Boland RA, Lin CS, Engel S, Kiernan MC. Adaptation of motor function after spinal cord injury: Novel insights into spinal shock. Brain. 2011;**134**(Pt 2):495–505. DOI: 10.1093/brain/awq289

[68] Popa C, Popa F, Grigorean VT, Onose G, Sandu AM, Popescu M, Burnei G, Strambu V, Sinescu C. Vascular dysfunctions following spinal cord injury. Journal of Medicine and Life. 2010;**3**(3):275–285

[69] Bracken MB, Shepard MJ, Holford TR, Leo-Summers L, Aldrich EF, Fazl M, Fehlings M, Herr DL, Hitchon PW, Marshall LF, Nockels RP, Pascale V, PL Jr P, Piepmeier J, Sonntag VK, Wagner F, Wilberger JE, Winn HR, Young W. Administration of methylprednisolone for 24 or 48 hours or tirilazad mesylate for 48 hours in the treatment of acute spinal cord injury. Results of the Third National Acute Spinal Cord Injury Randomized Controlled Trial. National Acute Spinal Cord Injury Study. JAMA. 1997;**277**(20):1597–1604

[70] Fehlings MG, Vaccaro A, Wilson JR, Singh A, Cadotte D W, JS H, Aarabi B, Shaffrey C, Dvorak M, Fisher C, Arnold P, EM M, Lewis S, Rampersaud R. Early versus delayed decompression for traumatic cervical spinal cord injury: Results of the Surgical Timing in Acute Spinal Cord Injury Study (STASCIS). PLoS One. 2012;**7**(2):e32037. DOI: 10.1371/journal.pone.0032037

[71] Vaccaro AR, Lambrechts MJ, Karamian BA, Canseco JA, Oner C, Benneker LM, Bransford R, Kandziora F, Shanmuganathan R, El-Sharkawi M, Kanna R, Joaquim A, Schnake K, Kepler CK, Schroeder GD. AO spine upper cervical injury classification international members. Global Validation of the AO Spine Upper Cervical Injury Classification. Spine (Philadelphia, Pennsylvania 1976). 2022;**47**(22):1541–1548. DOI: 10.1097/BRS.0000000000004429

[72] Karamian BA, Schroeder GD, Lambrechts MJ, Canseco JA, Oner C, Vialle E, Rajasekaran S, Dvorak MR, Benneker LM, Kandziora F, Schnake K, Kepler CK, Vaccaro AR; AO Spine Subaxial Classification Group Members. An international validation of the AO spine subaxial injury classification system. European Spine Journal. 2023;**32**(1):46–54. DOI: 10.1007/s00586-022-07467-6

[73] Radmard M, Tafazolimoghadam A, Amoah AA, Lakhani DA, Azad TD,

Bydon A, Yousem DM. Occipital condyle fractures revisited. Emergency Radiology. 2025;**32**(5):709–717. DOI: 10.1007/s10140-024-02303-4

[74] Cirak B, Akpinar G, Palaoglu S. Traumatic occipital condyle fractures. Neurosurgical Review. 2000;**23**(3):161–164. DOI: 10.1007/pl00011949

[75] Musbahi O, Khan AHA, Anwar MO, Chaudery H, Ali AM, Montgomery AS. Immobilisation in occipital condyle fractures: A systematic review. Clinical Neurology and Neurosurgery. 2018;**173**:130–139. DOI: 10.1016/j.clineuro.2018.08.013

[76] Hacking C, Deng F, Anderson and Montesano classification of occipital condyle fractures. Radiopaedia.org. DOI: 10.53347/rID-87202 [Accessed: 2025-October-26]

[77] Rief M, Zoidl P, Zajic P, Heschl S, Orlob S, Silbernagel G, Metnitz P, Puchwein P, Prause G. Atlanto-occipital dislocation in a patient presenting with out-of-hospital cardiac arrest: A case report and literature review. Journal of Medical Case Reports. 2019;**13**(1):44. DOI: 10.1186/s13256-018-1926-2

[78] Fard SA, Avila MJ, Johnstone CM, Patel AS, Walter CM, Skoch J, Sattarov KV, Baaj AA. Prognostic factors in traumatic atlanto-occipital dislocation. Journal of Clinical Neuroscience. 2016;**33**:63–68. DOI: 10.1016/j.jocn.2016.05.021

[79] Hacking C, Worsley C, Bell D. Traynelis classification of atlanto-occipital dislocations. Radiopaedia.org. DOI: 10.53347/rID-86945 [Accessed: 2025-October-26]

[80] Kumar A, Onggo J, Fon LH, Oh J. Direct fixation of C1 jefferson fracture using C1 lateral mass screws: A case report. International Journal of Spine Surgery. 2019;**13**(4):345–349. DOI: 10.14444/6047

[81] Agrawal R, Knipe H, Deng F, et al. Jefferson fracture. Reference article. Radiopaedia.org. DOI: 10.53347/rID-1534 [Accessed: 2025-October-26]

[82] Jones J, Gaillard F, Karuppannan J K, et al. Odontoid fracture. Reference article. Radiopaedia.org. DOI: 10.53347/rID-6370 [Accessed: 2025-October-26]

[83] Nourbakhsh A, Hanson ZC. Odontoid fractures: A standard review of current concepts and treatment recommendations. Journal of the American Academy of Orthopaedic Surgeons. 2022;**30**(6):e561–e572. DOI: 10.5435/JAAOS-D-21-00165

[84] Pepin JW, Hawkins RJ. Traumatic spondylolisthesis of the axis: Hangman's fracture. Clinical Orthopaedics and Related Research. 1981;**157**:1338

[85] Li XF, Dai LY, Lu H, Chen XD. A systematic review of the management of hangman's fractures. European Spine Journal. 2006;**15**(3):257–269. DOI: 10.1007/s00586-005-0918-2

[86] Goel A, Yap J, Hacking C, et al. Levine and Edwards classification of hangman (C2) fractures. Reference article. Radiopaedia.org. DOI: 10.53347/rID-35440 [Accessed: 2025-October-26]

[87] Feuchtbaum E, Buchowski J, Zebala L. Subaxial cervical spine trauma. Current Reviews in Musculoskeletal Medicine. 2016;**9**(4):496–504. DOI: 10.1007/s12178-016-9377-0

[88] Goel A, Molinari A, Hacking C, et al. Allen and Ferguson classification of subaxial cervical spine

injuries. Radiopaedia.org. DOI: 10.53347/rID-35493 [Accessed: 2025-October-26]

[89] Mainali S, Knipe H, Deng F, et al. Subaxial cervical spine injury classification. Radiopaedia.org. DOI: 10.53347/rID-66874 [Accessed: 2025-October-26]

[90] Robertson P, Zheng A, Hacking C, et al. Thoracolumbar injury classification and severity score (TLICS). Radiopaedia.org. DOI: 10.53347/rID-30250 [Accessed: 2025-October-26]

[91] Schubert R, Knipe H, Campos A, et al. Three column concept of spinal fractures. Radiopaedia.org. DOI: 10.53347/rID-15488 [Accessed: 2025-October-26]

[92] Vaccaro AR, Oner C, Kepler CK, Dvorak M, Schnake K, Bellabarba C, Reinhold M, Aarabi B, Kandziora F, Chapman J, Shanmuganathan R, Fehlings M, Vialle L. AOSpine spinal cord injury & trauma knowledge forum. AOSpine thoracolumbar spine injury classification system: Fracture description, neurological status, and key modifiers. Spine (Philadelphia, Pennsylvania 1976). 2013;**38**(23):2028–2037. DOI: 10.1097/BRS.0b013e3182a8a381

[93] Bydon M, Fredrickson V, De la Garza-ramos R, Li Y, RA Jr L, Trost GR, Gokaslan ZL. Sacral fractures. Neurosurgical Focus. 2014;**37**(1):E12. DOI: 10.3171/2014.5.FOCUS1474

[94] Skalski M, Walizai T, Gaillard F, et al. Classification of sacral fractures. Radiopaedia.org. DOI: 10.53347/rID-23212 [Accessed: 2025-October-26]

[95] Vaccaro AR, Schroeder GD, Divi SN, Kepler CK, Kleweno CP, Krieg JC, Wilson JR, Holstein JH, Kurd MF, Firoozabadi R, Vialle LR, Oner FC, Kandziora F, Chapman JR, Schnake KJ, Benneker LM, Dvorak MF, Rajasekaran S, Vialle EN, Joaquim AF, El-Sharkawi MM, Dhakal GR, Popescu EC, Kanna RM, Muijs SPJ, Tee JW, Bellabarba C. Description and reliability of the AOSpine sacral classification system. Journal of Bone and Joint Surgery. 2020;**102**(16):1454–1463. DOI: 10.2106/JBJS.19.01153

[96] Tavolaro C, Agel J, Vincent M, Dhillon E, Jung E, Zhou H. Post-operative follow-up care after acute spinal trauma: What is the reality? Brain and Spine. 2022;**2**:100905. DOI: 10.1016/j.bas.2022.100905.

[97] Smits AJ, Deunk J, Stadhouder A, Altena MC, Kempen DHR, Bloemers FW. Is postoperative bracing after pedicle screw fixation of spine fractures necessary? Study protocol of the ORNOT study: A randomised controlled multicentre trial. BMJ Open. 2018;**8**(1):e019596. DOI: 10.1136/bmjopen-2017-019596

[98] Braxton EE. Postoperative anesthesia and care pathways in ERAS for spine surgery. Seminars in Spine Surgery. 2025;**37**(3):101187. DOI: 10.1016/j.semss.2025.101187

Chapter 5

Diagnosis and Management of Calcaneal Fractures: Current Strategies

Sedeek M. Mosaid, Ashok Marudanayagam, Paul Lee, Yousif Jihad and Rizwan Shahid

Abstract

Calcaneal fractures represent the most prevalent type of tarsal fractures, comprising up to 75% of all foot fractures. The injuries tend to be related to high-energy trauma. The complex three-dimensional anatomy, multiple classification systems, and condition of the soft tissue envelope make the diagnosis and treatment of these fractures challenging in the affected patient. This chapter provides an updated review of the epidemiology, anatomy, and mechanisms of injury, as well as a detailed discussion of the classification of calcaneal fractures. The various treatment options, including nonoperative treatment, percutaneous treatment, open reduction, and internal fixation via extended lateral, sinus tarsi, and medial approaches, are discussed in detail. The use of subtalar arthroscopy and primary arthrodesis is also reviewed in the context of fracture patterns and patient-specific factors. Postoperative care, with an emphasis on early mobilisation and weight-bearing, is reviewed, with new data supporting an accelerated functional rehabilitation. In conclusion, the successful management of calcaneal fractures depends on an accurate assessment of the patient, meticulous management, and a proper choice of surgical technique, as well as a judicious decision-making process that is tailored to the patient's specific needs. The future of calcaneal fracture management will require higher-level evidence and the incorporation of emerging new technologies.

Keywords: calcaneal fractures, subtalar joint, open reduction and internal fixation (ORIF), minimally invasive fixation, arthroscopy, subtalar arthrodesis, postoperative rehabilitation

1. Introduction

Calcaneal fractures account for as much as 75% of all foot fractures and 1%–2% of all fractures. They are more common in men and individuals working in industrial occupations [1]. The incidence of these fractures peaks between 20 and 29 years of age in men and between 60 and 70 years in women [1].

Calcaneal fractures present many challenges for the surgeon. The complex bony anatomy and joint mechanics of the many tarsal bones, as well as the relatively delicate enveloping soft tissues, all contribute to the complexity of managing these fractures [2]. While several classification systems, surgical approaches, and postoperative protocols have been proposed, they have not gained universal acceptance, and the management of calcaneal fractures remains a subject of ongoing debate despite considerable progress in both diagnostic techniques and treatment options. In this regard, advancement towards a definitive management approach has been hindered by a lack of standardisation in fracture evaluation and classification [2].

Note: Böhler angle (see **Figure 1**) and Gissane angle (see **Figure 2**) will be discussed in Section 6 'Assessment'.

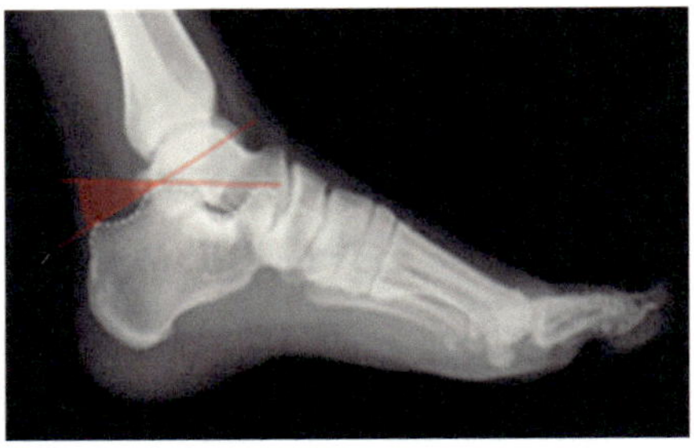

Figure 1.
Normal Böhler angle. Case courtesy of Leonardo Lustosa, Radiopaedia.org, rID: 94702.

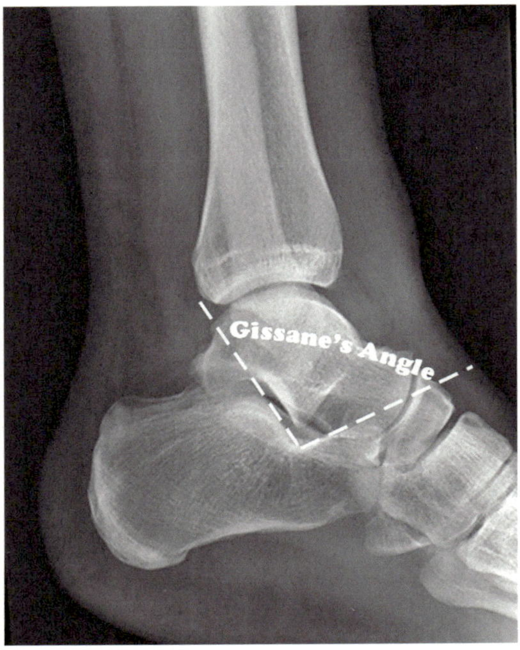

Figure 2.
Normal Gissane angle. Case courtesy of Samir Benoudina, Radiopaedia.org, rID: 40056.

2. Anatomy

A detailed understanding of calcaneal fracture anatomy is critical for rationalising the surgical approach. The anatomy of the calcaneus is complicated by the bone's three-dimensional (3D) form and its articulation with both the talus and the cuboid [3]. The calcaneus is the foot's largest bone, possessing a superior surface marked by three distinct articular facets: the posterior, middle, and anterior facets [4]. The sustentaculum tali, a notable bony ledge on the medial side, supports the neck of the talus [4].

The posterior facet, which is the most prominent, has an oval configuration, is convex in profile, and slopes distally and slightly laterally at approximately 45° in the sagittal orientation [4]. This facet is separated from the middle and anterior facets by the calcaneal sulcus, which delineates the medial edge of the tarsal canal and the lateral aspect of the sinus tarsi [4, 5]. The sinus tarsi, manifesting as a canal-like depression, comprises the anterior and middle facets as well as the talar sulcus and contains the anterior and posterior interosseous ligaments bridging the talus and calcaneus [4, 5].

The middle facet is characteristically concave, in contrast to the flat profile of the anterior facet. Notably, in around 20% of calcanei, the middle facet is fused with the anterior facet. The anterior process of the calcaneus exhibits a biconcave surface that interfaces with the cuboid, operating as a saddle joint and contributing to Chopart's midtarsal joint complex. This structure functions as a robust support for the lateral column of the foot [5,6].

The subtalar joint works closely with the ankle joint and affects distal foot articulations. It is a mitred hinge between the talus and the calcaneus, with a single axis that runs from medial to lateral at 16° to the sagittal plane and 42° above the horizontal plane [7]. This joint complex facilitates substantial inversion and eversion movements of the hindfoot, which are important for shock absorption at heel strike [7].

The lateral surface of the calcaneus is flat and ideal for internal fixation, but limited soft tissue coverage challenges wound healing. The medial wall is close to the posterior tibial neurovascular bundle, whose branches restrict surgical access [1, 8]. The sustentaculum tali is the most stable part of the calcaneus and relies on supporting tendons to maintain its anatomical position in most fractures [1, 8].

The medial side of the calcaneus receives its blood supply from perforating branches of the posterior tibial artery. The lateral calcaneal artery, which may arise from either the posterior tibial or the peroneal artery, supplies most of the lateral side [9].

A cadaveric study found that 10% of the blood supply stems from the sinus tarsi artery [9].

3. Mechanisms of calcaneal fracture

The classic mechanism of injury involves a high-energy axial load on the heel that drives the talus into the calcaneus. This results in two fracture lines because of a combination of shear and compression forces [10, 11]. Shear force divides the calcaneus into medial and lateral parts, while compression force divides it into anterior and posterior parts. The fracture line can extend medially and involve the middle facet [10, 11].

4. Common causes of calcaneal fracture

4.1 Falls from a height

Falling from a height, such as from a ladder or roof, is a leading cause of calcaneal fractures. Individuals who work in occupations or engage in activities that put them at risk for falls from heights are at an increased risk of sustaining such injuries [10, 11].

4.2 Motor vehicle accidents

Vehicle collisions can have a significant impact on the calcaneus. Subjecting the foot to crushing or direct impact forces can result in calcaneal fractures. These types of fractures are more common in high-speed collisions [11, 12].

4.3 Sports-related injuries

Some sports carry a greater chance of experiencing serious foot injuries, including calcaneal fractures. Athletes participating in high-contact sports, such as football, basketball, and gymnastics, are at a higher risk of sustaining these injuries [11].

5. Classification

Calcaneus fractures can be divided into extra-articular and intra-articular types, with extra-articular fractures making up 25%–40% and intra-articular fractures constituting 60%–75% [13,14].

Extra-articular fractures of the calcaneus are further classified based on their location in the anterior process, sustentaculum tali, and calcaneal tuberosity [13, 14]. The Beavis classification system categorises calcaneal tuberosity fractures by morphology. A type I or 'sleeve' fracture is an avulsion of the Achilles tendon with a small piece of cortical bone from the tuberosity. Type II or 'beak' fractures have oblique fracture lines extending posteriorly from the highest point of the posterior facet. Type III or 'infrabursal' fractures are avulsion fractures in the middle of the tuberosity [15].

Intra-articular fractures of the calcaneus (see **Figures 3** and **4**) can be categorised using either the Essex-Lopresti or Sanders classification systems (see **Figures 5–11**). The Essex-Lopresti method relies on lateral radiographs to identify fracture lines [14]. Here, the main fracture line passes through the posterior facet. Such fractures are identified as either tongue-type or depressed, depending on whether the secondary fracture line that exits posteriorly passes through or below the calcaneal tubercle. The tongue-type fragment is characterised by the attachment of the posterior tuberosity, while the joint-depressed fragment lacks this feature. Although the type of fracture influences the treatment approach, it does not affect the prognosis [14, 16].

The Sanders classification system employs coronal computed tomography (CT) scans to assess the number of articular fragments in the broadest section of the posterior facet, specifically at the level of the sustentaculum tali. Type I fractures are characterised by being nondisplaced or having less than 2 mm of articular

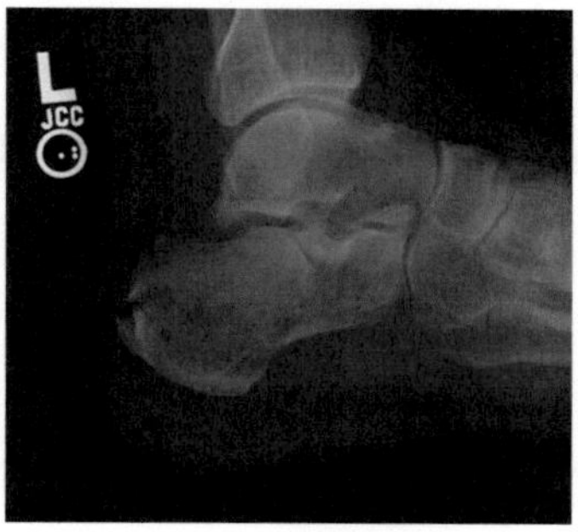

Figure 3.
Left intra-articular calcaneal fracture with decreased Böhler angle. Case courtesy of The Radswiki, Radiopaedia.org, rID: 11269.

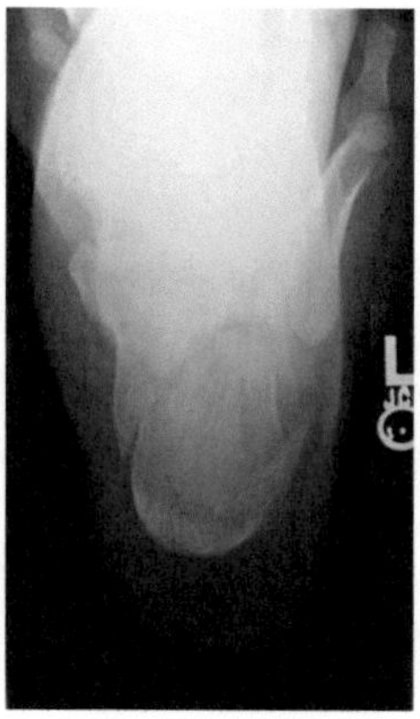

Figure 4.
Axial view of left intra-articular calcaneal fracture with decreased Böhler angle.Case courtesy of The Radswiki, Radiopaedia.org, rID: 11269.

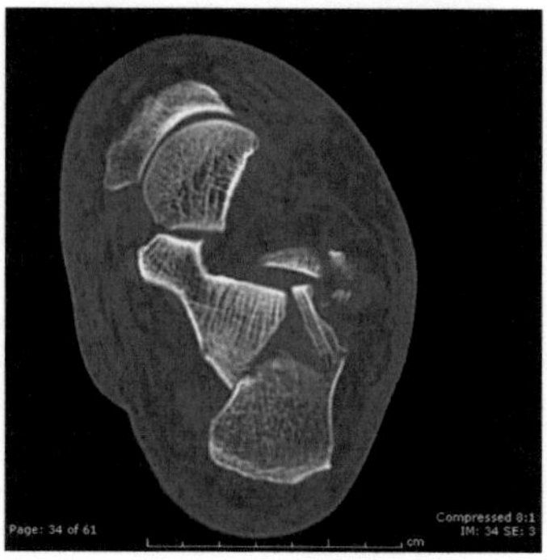

Figure 5.
Sanders type IIA fracture involving the lateral aspect of the posterior facet of the calcaneus.Case courtesy of Matt Skalski, Radiopaedia.org, rID: 27027.

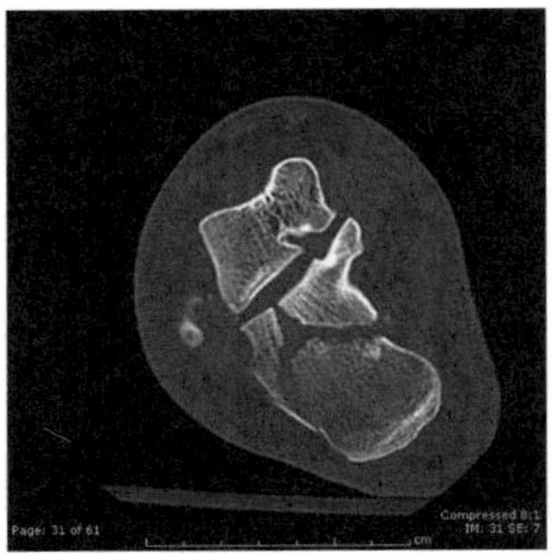

Figure 6.
Sanders type IIB fracture with a fracture line extending into the middle posterior facet of the right calcaneus. Case courtesy of Matt Skalski, Radiopaedia.org, rID: 26988.

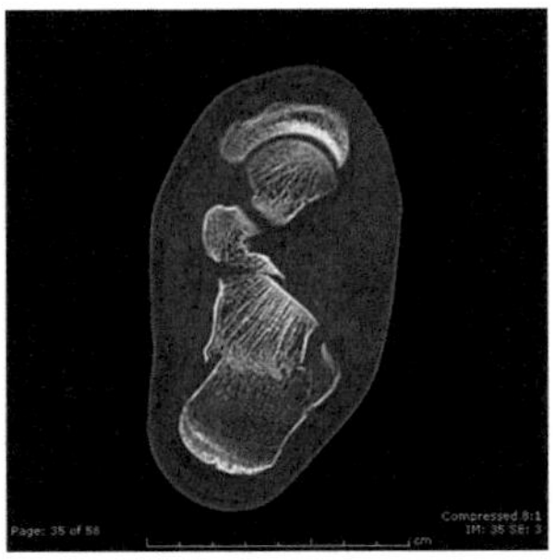

Figure 7.
Sanders type IIC fracture coursing through the most lateral aspect of the posterior facet of the calcaneus. Case courtesy of Matt Skalski, Radiopaedia.org, rID: 27028.

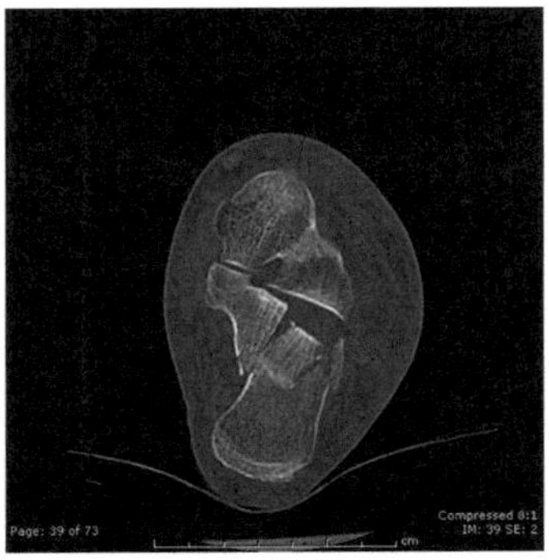

Figure 8.
Type IIIAB fracture detailing two primary fracture lines extending through the lateral and central aspects of the posterior facet of the calcaneus. Case courtesy of Matt Skalski, Radiopaedia.org, rID: 27029.

displacement, irrespective of the number of fracture lines or fragments. Type II fractures (see **Figures 5–7**) are displaced two-part fractures of the posterior facet. They are categorised into three main subtypes: A, B, and C, depending on the location of the primary fracture line from lateral to medial [14, 17]. Type III fractures (see **Figures 8–10**) involve displaced three-part fractures with an associated central

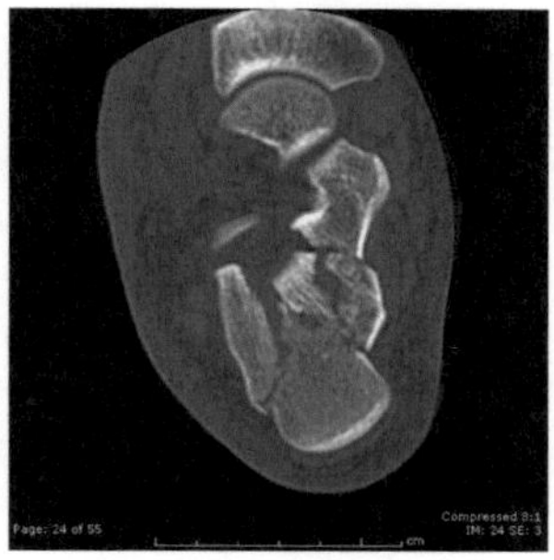

Figure 9.
Type IIIAC fracture, detailing two primary fracture lines extending through the lateral and medial aspects of the posterior facet of the calcaneus.Case courtesy of Matt Skalski, Radiopaedia.org, rID: 27030.

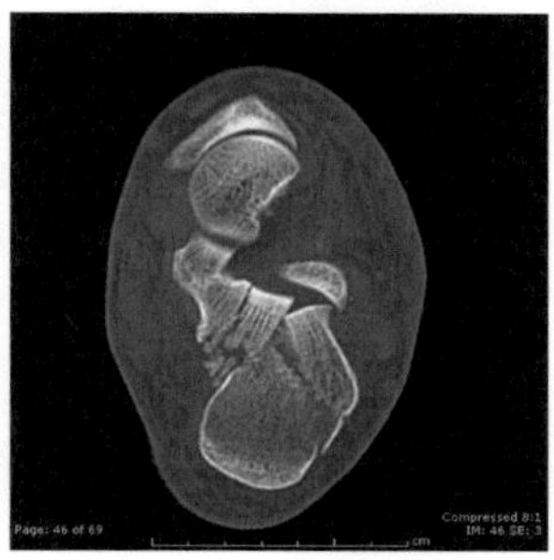

Figure 10.
Type IIIBC fracture detailing two primary fracture lines through the central and medial aspects of the posterior facet of the calcaneus. Case courtesy of Matt Skalski, Radiopaedia.org, rID: 27031.

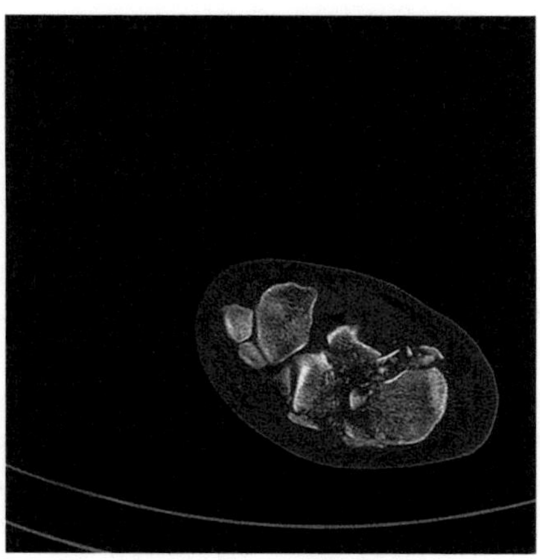

Figure 11.
Type IV Sanders fracture. There is evidence of intra-articular, severely comminuted fractures of right calcaneus. Case courtesy of Naqibullah Foladi, Radiopaedia.org, rID: 90179.

depression, with subtypes determined by the location of the fracture lines extending into the posterior facet. Type IV fractures (see **Figure 11**) are comminuted intra-articular fractures consisting of four or more parts, with three or more fracture lines reaching the joint, often accompanied by significant displacement [14, 17].

6. Assessment

Calcaneal fractures are usually caused by high-energy trauma. Patients with these injuries should be evaluated and treated following the Advanced Trauma and Life Support guidelines, which are constantly being updated. There is a 10% incidence of high thoracic and lumbar spine injuries, as well as contralateral calcaneal fractures. Notably, there is a correlation with other foot injuries and talar neck fractures, which also occur in 10% of cases. These injuries are generally seen in high-energy trauma cases [1, 18].

Assessing the fracture patient's medical history, lifestyle habits, and daily routines is vital, as these factors can influence outcomes. For example, vascular disease, past infections in the hindfoot, and smoking play a role in determining overall results. When multiple risk factors are present, the relative risk of wound complications increases cumulatively [1, 19].

Appropriate clinical examination of hindfoot fractures is important because the soft tissue envelope is delicate and requires precise treatment. The degree of displacement and soft tissue injury is directly related to the force at the time of injury. In severe cases, open fractures can occur; in milder cases, the medial spike of the superomedial fragment can breach the skin and create a small medial puncture wound. A high degree of suspicion is necessary to avoid missing this type of fracture [2, 6, 20].

Calcaneal fractures are painful; this pain is sharp and localised to the heel. It gets worse with weight-bearing as the fractured calcaneus is subjected to stress. The pain level can vary depending on the type and severity of the fracture [11]. Swelling around the heel and side of the foot is another common symptom in calcaneal fractures. If the patient is evaluated more than six hours after the injury, the swelling is generally so pronounced that skin creases are no longer visible. In some cases, the swelling can be so extreme that blisters develop; these may be intradermal (clear fluid) or full-thickness (serosanguineous fluid). Compartment syndrome should be considered, especially in high-energy or crush injuries [6, 21]. The calcaneal compartment, which includes the quadratus plantae and lateral plantar nerves, is most commonly affected in calcaneal fractures. High pressures in the compartment can cause ischaemic damage and often lead to claw toes, sensory abnormalities, stiffness, chronic pain, and atrophy [22, 23].

The recommended plain radiographs are lateral hindfoot, anteroposterior (AP) foot and ankle, and Harris axial heel. Lateral hindfoot images are essential for assessing calcaneus height, Böhler's angle (see **Figure 1**), and Gissane's angle (see **Figure 2**). They also show minor avulsion fractures in the anterior process or posterior tuberosity. Thus, this view is key for diagnosing a calcaneal fracture.

Böhler's angle is measured by the highest points of the anterior process, posterior facet, and tuberosity of the calcaneus. Normal values are 25°–40°. A reduction in this angle indicates depression or an intra-articular fracture. Gissane's angle is measured by the downward and upward slopes of the superior calcaneal surface. Normal values are 130°–145°. Any deviation from this range indicates articular involvement [24, 25]. Gissane's angle increases solely when the posterior facet detaches from the superomedial fragment. If the fracture and depression occur only in the lateral half of the facet, a 'double density' sign appears. In such instances, Böhler's angle remains unchanged [6, 24]. Typically, the depressed articular surface is rotated 90° to the rest of the joint surface. The lateral radiograph also helps determine whether the fracture is of the joint-depressed type or the tongue type [6, 24].

The AP radiograph shows that the fracture line may extend into the calcaneocuboid joint, along with any related midfoot issues.

Harris axial radiography helps evaluate the comminution of the lateral wall and the heel's position. Only the central section of the posterior articular facet is visible; the rest of the joint is obscured by overlapping structures, making this view unreliable for a complete assessment of the articular surface. Additionally, this view is challenging to obtain in acute cases due to pain [4, 6].

Broden's projection is a specialised oblique radiographic view of the calcaneus, primarily used to evaluate the posterior facet of the subtalar joint after injury. It is particularly valuable for assessing intra-articular displacement and verifying articular reduction following operative fixation [25–27].

The patient is placed in the supine position, with the affected foot internally rotated 30°–40°. The X-ray beam is angled cephalad at varying angles (10°, 20°, 30°, and 40°) to visualise different portions of the posterior facet. Lower beam angles show the anterior part of the facet, while higher angles visualise its posterior aspect. Broden's projection remains helpful intraoperatively and in postoperative follow-up when CT is not feasible [25, 26, 28].

Fine-slice CT scans with multiplanar reconstructions are considered the gold standard for visualising calcaneal fractures. These scans are essential for classifying fracture patterns, making treatment decisions, and planning surgeries. CT scans can also evaluate the loss of normal foot contours [6, 17].

Coronal and transverse CT images are captured using 2-mm sections for accurate calcaneus assessment. The coronal images should be perpendicular to the posterior articular facet, while the transverse images should align parallel to the foot. Coronal images reveal the number and location of articular fragments. The calcaneal body is examined for any widening or shortening, and the tuberosity is checked for its position [6, 29, 30]. Transverse images also display lateral wall blowout, showing comminution of the sustentaculum and the calcaneocuboid joint surface. The anteroinferior posterior articular facet is best observed in these sections [6, 29, 30].

7. Treatment

Treatment options can be divided into emergent, nonoperative, minimally invasive open reduction with internal fixation (ORIF), standard ORIF, and primary arthrodesis procedures [2, 6]. These are detailed below.

7.1 Emergent procedures

Emergent procedures are necessary only when the soft tissue envelope is at risk, such as in cases of the foot developing compartment syndrome, an open fracture, or when displaced bone fragments severely tent the skin [2,6].

Open calcaneal fractures are rarer than closed ones. Standard procedures for their treatment include irrigation and debridement of the open area, typically a small puncture wound on the medial side caused by the superomedial fragment's spike. The wound is then covered with a standard dressing, a vacuum-type dressing, or temporarily closed with skin substitutes [31, 32]. An external fixator may be used for tibiometatarsal transfixation; alternatively, a three-point distractor can be placed with pins in the talus, calcaneal tuberosity, and cuboid. After 48 to 72 hours, a second evaluation with repeat debridement is conducted to determine the type of soft tissue coverage needed. Standard osteosynthesis is usually performed after the soft tissue has recovered, typically within 10 to 14 days, but this procedure can be delayed by up to 3 weeks to allow for stabilisation. If coverage is insufficient for closure but the overall condition is good, early osteosynthesis might be supplemented with a local or free-flap procedure to ensure complete wound closure. This approach reduces infection rates and enables early functional after-treatment [6, 32, 33].

When compartment syndrome is confirmed, including pressures exceeding 30 mmHg or within 10–30 mmHg of the diastolic pressure, an urgent fasciotomy becomes necessary. This procedure involves making a medial incision of about 6 cm in length, beginning 4 cm in front of the heel and 3 cm above the foot's plantar surface. The medial compartment is accessed, and the abductor hallucis muscle is lifted until the medial intermuscular septum is visible. The fascia is then opened to release the deep calcaneal compartment. During this procedure, the lateral plantar nerve is vulnerable as it is located just to the side of the medial septum. Depending on the injury, the dorsal compartments may also be released. In patients with multiple traumas, this procedure is followed by indirect reduction, K-wiring, and external fixation. For those with isolated calcaneal fractures, the release of the compartment may be followed by standard osteosynthesis [6, 20, 22, 23].

When bone fragments are severely displaced and tented against the skin, they can cause full-thickness skin death. The surgeon must identify any such areas during the first examination of the foot. This type of skin damage can develop rapidly and often presents a significant challenge to effective management. These displaced fragments should be treated using a percutaneous reduction method, along with temporary external and K-wire fixation, to allow the soft tissues to stabilise before proceeding with a formal open reduction. Many such calcaneus fractures are associated with significant soft tissue compromise [6, 34, 35].

7.2 Nonoperative procedures

Nonoperative management is typically preferred for nondisplaced fractures or those that are only slightly displaced. This approach is often advised for extra-articular fractures with fragment sizes smaller than 1 cm and displacements of less than 2 mm, provided the Achilles tendon remains intact. It is also suitable for Sanders type I intra-articular fractures [6, 36, 37].

Nonoperative procedures are also utilised when there are specific local or general reasons to avoid surgery. Conditions that contraindicate ORIF include severe neurovascular insufficiency, poorly managed insulin-dependent diabetes mellitus, patient noncompliance (such as due to substance abuse), and severe systemic disorders that involve immunodeficiency or a generally poor prognosis. Additionally, the condition of the soft tissue being questionable, such as in cases of significant blistering or extensive swelling, contraindicates surgical procedures [2, 20, 35]. Advanced age alone is not a reason to avoid surgery, as positive outcomes can be achieved in active patients over 65 years old. Rather, treatment is customised based on the patient's functional needs, existing health conditions, and level of compliance [38, 39].

7.3 Minimally invasive options

Using minimally invasive techniques to fix calcaneal fractures can greatly minimise the risk of soft tissue problems. Many experts recommend percutaneous reduction and screw fixation for extra-articular and simple intra-articular fractures where the posterior facet is displaced as a whole, such as in Sanders type IIC fractures [40, 41]. These methods can also be applied to intra-articular fractures with a single displaced fracture line across the subtalar joint (i.e., Sanders types IIA and IIB), provided that the articular reduction is properly monitored using subtalar arthroscopy or 3D fluoroscopy [42, 43]. However, attempting percutaneous reduction and fixation without ensuring adequate control of the reduction, regardless of the fracture type, can lead to poor reduction and fixation failure [44, 45].

Percutaneous screw fixation, which involves inserting screws through small incisions directly into the fractured calcaneal segments, is one of two standard percutaneous techniques [11, 46]. This minimally invasive approach aims to provide stability and alignment without the need for large incisions. It is particularly beneficial for fractures suitable for this method, offering advantages such as reduced soft tissue damage and potentially quicker postoperative recovery [11, 46].

The second standard technique, external fixation, involves using external frames to maintain the alignment and stability of the fractured calcaneus. This technique is often used for complex fractures or when internal fixation is not suitable, as the external frame provides support and allows for controlled adjustments, enhancing overall stability. Although external fixation requires placing pins through the skin into the bone, it is beneficial in specific clinical situations [11, 47].

7.4 ORIF option

The aims of surgical intervention for calcaneal fractures include achieving bony union without infection and ensuring an early functional return (see **Figure 12**). Operative fixation prioritises heel height restoration and varus correction, tuberosity fragment control, subtalar joint reconstruction, medial and lateral wall reconstruction, and the protection of tendon and neurovascular structures [1].

Pre-operative preparation includes strict skin monitoring, elevation, and ice application [1, 6]. Apart from this, the timing of surgery is critical. Early surgery within three days of injury increases the risk of wound breakdown and necrosis. Osteosynthesis for closed calcaneal fractures is usually performed one to two weeks after injury, when haematoma and swelling have decreased and skin blisters have healed [48]. If percutaneous fixation is planned, surgery should not be delayed more than seven days after injury because percutaneous reduction reportedly becomes more difficult beyond that time [40]. Generally, if more than three weeks have passed since injury, nonoperative management is the best option because the fragments have likely already started to consolidate [20, 36, 49].

Sanders recommends looking for a positive wrinkle test. This test involves direct palpation of the skin over the lateral aspect of the calcaneus and visual evaluation of this area when the patient dorsiflexes and everts the foot [20]. If skin wrinkling is seen and no pitting oedema is present, the test is considered positive, and surgery can be performed [20].

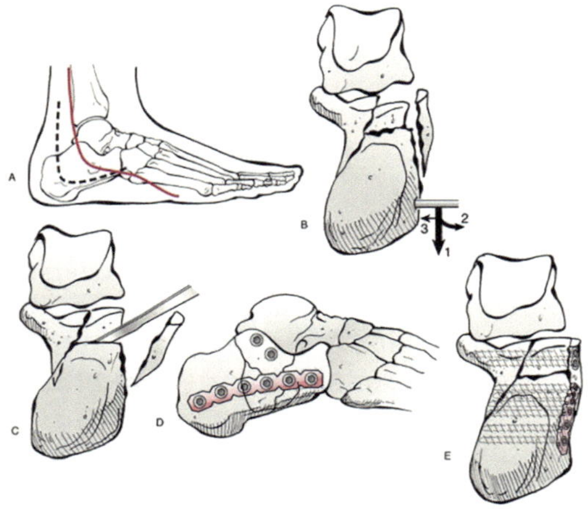

Figure 12.
The extensile lateral L-shaped incision used in open reduction and internal fixation (ORIF) of calcaneal fractures. The vertical limb is placed between the fibula and Achilles tendon, and the horizontal limb extends along the lateral border of the calcaneus. TeachMeOrthopedics. (2024) Fractures and dislocations of the foot.

Several surgical approaches have been outlined for managing calcaneal fractures, including the medial, sustentacular, sinus tarsi, and extended lateral exposures. Among these, the extended lateral approach is widely utilised, as it provides excellent visualisation of the posterior facet and is particularly advantageous in addressing complex fractures with marked displacement and multiple intra-articular extensions involving the subtalar joint [39, 50].

7.4.1 Extended lateral approach

This technique provides excellent visualisation of the comminuted lateral wall, fractured posterior facet, sinus tarsi, and anterior process, including the calcaneocuboidal joint. However, it necessitates meticulous handling of soft tissues, involving the elevation of a full-thickness fasciocutaneous flap from the lateral calcaneal wall and careful mobilisation of the peroneal tendons within their sheath while respecting the path of the sural nerve and the lateral calcaneal artery [2, 50]. The skin incision is L-shaped on the lateral side of the heel, extending between the lateral malleolus and the posterior and inferior borders of the heel [2]. Considering the blood supply to the lateral heel via the lateral calcaneal artery and the sural nerve's path, the incision is not precisely midway between the lateral malleolus and the foot's edge. Rather, it is directed more towards the sole and the Achilles tendon's border. This approach was developed using a full-thickness flap [50–52]. The peroneal tendons are mobilised within their sheath and gently retracted with a Penrose drain to prevent postoperative adhesions. After exposing the subtalar joint and identifying the primary fracture line at Gissane's angle, the reduction of the tuberosity fragment can often be facilitated with an axially placed 6.5 mm Schanz screw [2, 35]. Alternatively, a 4.5–5.5 mm screw can be inserted from the lateral side [2]. This manoeuvre also enhances visualisation and facilitates the elevation of the depressed posterior facet fragment. The fractured posterior facet is sequentially reduced from the medial to the lateral side. The reconstructed posterior facet is then aligned with the tuberosity and anterior process fragments and secured with additional K-wires [2].

7.4.2 Sinus tarsi approach

The sinus tarsi approach has become a recognised technique for managing intra-articular calcaneal fractures, especially displaced Sanders type II injuries and selected type III fractures. The technique is performed through a smaller skin incision, approximately 4–6 cm, from the distal fibula to the fourth metatarsal base [53, 54]. Dissection through the sinus tarsi, accompanied by careful elevation of the extensor digitorum brevis, allows for direct access to the subtalar joint's posterior facet with minimal soft tissue disruption. The depressed fragments are elevated, calcaneal height and alignment are re-established, and fixation with low-profile plates or screws is performed. A principal benefit of this approach is a measurable reduction in wound complications relative to the extensile lateral incision [53, 54].

The sinus tarsi approach typically decreases operative time, spares the periosteal blood supply, and enables earlier postoperative mobilisation. Furthermore, the technique affords a direct view of the posterior facet, a crucial element in attaining an accurate reduction [35, 55]. Nevertheless, it has certain limitations. Reduced exposure hinders the optimal management of severely comminuted injuries, such as Sanders type IV fractures. Precise, anatomically relevant manipulation of the tuberosity fragment, along with the correction of potential malalignment in the lateral wall, becomes technically more challenging with this approach, and the learning curve can be steep, with a risk of malreduction for less-experienced surgeons [56, 57].

Accordingly, patient selection should be restricted to those with displaced intra-articular fractures characterised by moderate comminution, posterior facet depression, or anticipated complications related to extended incisional length (e.g., patients with heavy tobacco use or poorly controlled diabetes). In such selected cases, the depressed posterior facet fragment is identified, elevated, and provisionally fixed with K-wires. Definitive fixation is then performed to restore Böhler's angle, Gissane's angle, and overall calcaneal morphology [58, 59].

7.4.3 Medial approach

The medial approach has been used for simple two-part fractures, extra-articular fractures, and medial wall blowout. Generally, a lateral incision is needed to reduce the joint. This incision is horizontal or lazy S-shaped, 8–10 cm long, between the medial malleolus tip and the sole. The neurovascular bundle is identified and retracted, the abductor hallucis longus muscle is pulled down, and the flexor hallucis longus tendon is identified [60, 61]. The sustentacular fragment is fully exposed, and the medial facet is directly controlled. The tuberosity fragment is indirectly reduced by applying axial traction to the sustentacular fragment and the anterior process if it is detached from the main tuberosity fragment. After temporary K-wire fixation, final fixation is performed with a small plate in an anti-glide position [60, 61]. The advantages of this approach include fewer wounds and infection-related complications. However, this approach is less popular now, partly because it does not allow direct visualisation of the subtalar joint [58].

7.5 Subtalar arthroscopy in calcaneal fracture fixation

Subtalar arthroscopy is gaining popularity as an adjunct to calcaneal fracture surgery, as it enables direct visualisation of the posterior facet and assessment of articular reduction, helping detect any remaining step-offs or gaps after reduction and allowing for precise screw placement to minimise joint penetration and maximise fixation. Arthroscopy also allows for the removal of trapped fragments, the washing out of haemarthrosis, and the assessment of subtalar cartilage injuries, which are often missed with open or percutaneous techniques. Standard anterolateral and posterolateral portals are used for visualisation and can also be used for shavers and other arthroscopic instruments [58, 62].

Despite its benefits, this technique can add to surgery time, has a steep learning curve, increases soft tissue swelling due to fluid introduction, and complicates setup. Nevertheless, overall, arthroscopically assisted fixation is a minimally invasive method that improves intraoperative precision and long-term functional outcomes in selected intra-articular calcaneal fractures [43, 63].

7.6 Plate fixation and defect filling

When the depressed section of the thalamus is elevated, it often leaves a bony defect due to the fragment being driven into the cancellous bone and the neutral triangle. The need to fill this defect, either with a bone graft from the same side's iliac crest or with bone substitutes, is debated. A bone graft has been shown to be unnecessary, as the 'neutral triangle' will fill with cancellous bone in eight weeks [64, 65].

However, a graft is recommended in unstable reductions. In cases of significant bone loss, such as open or comminuted fractures, bone substitute void fillers, like calcium sulphate–hydroxyapatite formulations, are helpful during the initial reconstruction phase. They maintain space and deliver local antibiotics, allowing for delayed definitive fixation [2, 64, 66].

The ideal plate has a low profile, and screws can be placed directly under the joint surface and across the calcaneus body for three-point fixation. Anatomically contoured plates allow for optimal screw placement [6].

Over the years, various plates have been recommended. Most studies indicate that stability can be achieved with a single lateral plate that mimics the anatomy of the calcaneus, supporting the tuberosity, the talocalcaneal portion, and the anterior process. Most modern plates are polyaxial. When using an interlocking plate, one or two conventional screws should be placed first to bring the plate closer to the bone, thereby enhancing stability through friction and preventing soft tissue impingement caused by plate protrusion [67].

The choice of plate type depends on the fracture's complexity and the quality of the bone. Non-locking plates may be sufficient for simple patterns, while highly comminuted or osteoporotic fractures benefit from locking plates that provide angular stability and lower wound complication rates [67–69].

7.7 Primary subtalar arthrodesis

Subtalar arthrodesis is an option for severely comminuted intra-articular calcaneal fractures, especially Sanders type IV fractures, where anatomical reconstruction of the posterior facet is not possible [1, 36]. This choice of modality is based on the high incidence of post-traumatic subtalar arthritis in this group (up to 71%) and the increased chance of needing secondary fusion after standard fixation or conservative management [70].

The surgical technique involves restoring the height and alignment of the calcaneus, removing any remaining cartilage, and using an autologous bone graft and lag screws for fixation, sometimes with the addition of a lateral plate [71].

Case series and reviews have demonstrated promising results with primary fusion, including high union rates (90%–100%), return-to-work rates of 75%–100%, and an average AOFAS (American Orthopaedic Foot and Ankle Society) score of 77.4. However, wound complications remain a concern. Additionally, despite the positive results, evidence from a randomised controlled trial suggests that primary fusion is not superior to ORIF, with only a small number of patients requiring delayed secondary arthrodesis after initial fixation [72]. Therefore, while primary subtalar arthrodesis is an option in some cases of severe comminution, experts recommend trying ORIF first and reserving arthrodesis for patients who later develop painful subtalar osteoarthritis [72].

8. Postoperative Care

Early postoperative management is centred around oedema control, wound care, and dressing changes. Ankle and subtalar range of motion is usually initiated after wound healing is stable to minimise stiffness and promote rapid functional recovery [73]. Postoperative management protocols commonly avoid weight-bearing or contact activities for 8–12 weeks in the immediate postoperative period. However, recent literature, including a 2018 systematic review and a 2025 meta-analysis, shows that early permissive/partial weight-bearing initiated in the first two to four weeks in selected, stably fixed fractures is safe, with no increased rates of loss of reduction or complications; additionally, it improves patient-reported outcomes and shortens the time to return to preinjury activities [74–76]. Cohort data on screws-only fixation also reveal no radiographic failures with early weight-bearing pathways when used in the setting of close clinical and radiographic follow-up [77]. Thus, a typical follow-up protocol includes a wound check approximately one week postoperatively, suture removal at two weeks, and then a progressive protocol for partial weight-bearing, directed by symptoms and interval radiographs [73, 75, 76].

9. Complications

Complications following calcaneal fractures are common, occurring with both operative and nonoperative management. The most common postoperative complication is superficial wound edge necrosis, which occurs in up to 14% of patients after the extended lateral approach and up to 27% of patients after the medial and lateral approach [6, 78]. Predictors of complications include smoking, obesity, open injury, and a time to surgery greater than two weeks. Superficial necrosis is most often treated conservatively with local wound care or negative pressure therapy; however, in some cases, flap coverage may be required. Deep infection is much less common but often requires radical debridement and prolonged antibiotic administration. In some cases, hardware removal and flap coverage are required, and chronic osteomyelitis may necessitate a subtotal calcanectomy [6, 19].

Nerve injuries are most common in the sural nerve and posterior tibial nerve, resulting in hypaesthesia or neuroma formation. Treatment is most often conservative, involving neuroma excision if symptomatic [2, 6].

Hardware-induced irritation is thought to be a cause of peroneal tendonitis, particularly if the peroneal tendon sheath was violated. In some cases, tenolysis and implant removal may be necessary [2, 6].

Malunion is a well-recognised complication of displaced calcaneal fractures, whether nonoperatively managed or incompletely reduced. Symptomatic malunion is characteristically disabling, leading to a combination of the following typical deformities: loss of calcaneal height, heel widening, varus or valgus malalignment, fibulocalcaneal impingement, and peroneal tendon subluxation or irritation [2, 6]. These conditions are typically associated with painful subtalar arthritis, and in more chronic or advanced cases, tibiotalar impingement or tilt with secondary ankle arthritis [2, 6].

Isolated subtalar arthrodesis alone can address post-traumatic arthritis pain but cannot correct the malunion or restore hindfoot alignment and function. Subtalar distraction bone block arthrodesis, to restore calcaneal height and unload tibiotalar impingement, was first described by Carr et al. and subsequently found to be a reliable technique for addressing this concern [79].

Romash [80] combined distraction arthrodesis with a corrective osteotomy along the original fracture line, achieving good outcomes in most cases.

The evolution of modern 3D CT planning has increased the accuracy of the above procedures. However, they remain salvage operations, intended to provide pain relief and functional improvement, and do not address the primary issues of foot mechanics. The outcomes emphasise the need to achieve an accurate index procedure reduction to avoid the cascade of complications resulting from malunion [2, 6, 81].

10. Conclusion

Calcaneal fractures remain among the most complex injuries in orthopaedic trauma, with outcomes closely tied to accurate assessment, meticulous technical application, and patient-specific decision-making. While advances in imaging, minimally invasive fixation, and early functional rehabilitation have refined management, no single strategy is universally applicable. The extended lateral approach continues to provide reliable exposure for complex patterns, but sinus tarsi and percutaneous techniques enable lower levels of soft tissue morbidity in selected cases. Primary subtalar arthrodesis and corrective salvage procedures are valuable in cases of severe comminution or malunion but highlight the importance of achieving anatomical reduction at the index surgery. Postoperative protocols increasingly support early mobilisation and permissive weight-bearing, reflecting a shift towards functionally oriented care. Future progress will depend on higher-level evidence to guide surgical indications, the implementation of advanced planning tools such as 3D imaging and patient-specific implants, and long-term functional studies. Ultimately, achieving the best results requires balancing surgical innovation with the fundamental principles of fracture care.

Author details

Sedeek M. Mosaid[1*], Ashok Marudanayagam[2], Paul Lee[2], Yousif Jihad[3] and Rizwan Shahid[4]

1 FRCS (Orth) (first author), Orthopaedic Specialty Doctor, Department of Trauma & Orthopaedics, United Lincolnshire Teaching Hospitals NHS Trust, Lincoln, United Kingdom

2 FRCS (Orth) Consultant Orthopaedic Surgeon Department of Trauma & Orthopaedics, United Lincolnshire Teaching Hospitals NHS Trust, Lincoln, United Kingdom

3 Resident Doctor, Department of Trauma & Orthopaedics, United Lincolnshire Hospitals NHS Trust, Lincoln, United Kingdom

4 Consultant Orthopaedic Surgeon Department of Trauma and Orthopaedics, United Lincolnshire Teaching Hospitals NHS Trust, Lincoln, United Kingdom

*Address all correspondence to: sedeeko2000@hotmail.com

References

[1] Razik A, Harris M, Trompeter A. Calcaneal fractures: Where are we now?. Strategies in Trauma and Limb Reconstruction. 2017;**13**:1–11. https://www.ncbi.nlm.nih.gov/pmc/articles/PMC5862705/

[2] Rammelt S, Zwipp H. Calcaneus fractures: Facts, controversies and recent developments. Injury. 2004;**35**:443–461

[3] Keener BJ, Sizensky JA. The anatomy of the calcaneus and surrounding structures. Foot and Ankle Clinics. 2005;**10**:413–424. DOI: 10.1016/j.fcl.2005.04.003

[4] Hall RL, Shereff MJ. Anatomy of the calcaneus. Clinical Orthopaedics and Related Research. 1993;**290**:27–35

[5] Sarrafian SK. Anatomy of the Foot and Ankle. Philadelphia: Lippincott; 1993

[6] Maskill JD, Bohay DR, Anderson JG. Calcaneus Fractures: A Review Article. Foot and Ankle Clinics. 2005;**10**: 463–489

[7] Inman VT. The Joints of the Ankle. Baltimore: Williams & Wilkins; 1976

[8] Epstein N, Chandran S, Chou L. Current concepts review: Intra-Articular fractures of the Calcaneus. Foot & Ankle International. 2012;**33**:79–86

[9] Andermahr J, Helling HJ, Rehm KE, Koebke J. The vascularization of the os calcaneum and the clinical consequences. Clinical Orthopaedics and Related Research. 1999;**363**: 212–218

[10] Galluzzo M, Greco F, Pietragalla M, Renzis AD, Carbone M, Zappia M, et al. Calcaneal fractures: Radiological and CT evaluation and classification systems. Acta Bio Medica: Atenei Parmensis. 2018;**89**:138. https://www.ncbi.nlm.nih.gov/labs/pmc/articles/PMC6179077/

[11] Chirayath A, Dhaniwala N, Kawde K. A Comprehensive Review on Managing Fracture Calcaneum by Surgical and Non-surgical Modalities. Cureus. 2024;**16**(2):e54786. DOI: 10.7759/cureus.54786.

[12] Benson E, Conroy C, Hoyt DB, Eastman AB, Pacyna S, Smith J, et al. Calcaneal fractures in occupants involved in severe frontal motor vehicle crashes. Accident; Analysis and Prevention. 2007;**39**:794–799. Available from: https://pubmed.ncbi.nlm.nih.gov/17250792/

[13] Box MW, Domingue GA, Werthmann NJ, Szatkowski JP, Riehl JT. Calcaneus Fractures. IntechOpen eBooks [Internet]. 2024. Available from: https://www.intechopen.com/chapters/89058

[14] Schepers T, Ginai AZ, van Lieshout EM, Patka P. Demographics of extra-articular calcaneal fractures: Including a review of the literature on treatment and outcome. Archives of Orthopaedic and Trauma Surgery. 2008;**128**:1099–1106. DOI: 10.1007/s00402-007-0517-2

[15] Lee SM, Huh SW, Chung JW, Kim DW, Kim YJ, Rhee SK. Avulsion fracture of the calcaneal tuberosity: Classification and its characteristics. Clinics in Orthopedic Surgery.

2012;**4**:134–138. Available from: https://www.ncbi.nlm.nih.gov/pubmed/22662299

[16] Schepers T, van Lieshout EMM, Ginai AZ, Mulder PGH, Heetveld MJ, Patka P. Calcaneal fracture classification: A comparative study. The Journal of Foot and Ankle Surgery. 2009;**48**:156–162. DOI: 10.1053/j.jfas.2008.11.00

[17] Sanders R, Fortin P, DiPasquale T, Walling A. Operative treatment in 120 displaced intraarticular calcaneal fractures: Results using a prognostic computed tomography scan classification. Clinical Orthopaedics and Related Research. 1993;**290**:87–95

[18] Kortbeek JB, Al Turki SA, Ali J, Antoine JA, Bouillon B, Brasel K, et al. Advanced trauma life support, 8th edition, the evidence for change. The Journal of Trauma. 2008;**64**:1638–1650

[19] Folk JW, Starr AJ, Early JS. Early wound complications of operative treatment of calcaneus fractures: Analysis of 190 fractures. Journal of Orthopaedic Trauma. 1999;**13**:369–372

[20] Sanders R. Displaced intra-articular fractures of the calcaneus. The Journal of Bone and Joint Surgery-American Volume. 2000;**82**:225–250

[21] Giordano CP, Koval KJ. Treatment of fracture blisters: A prospective study of 53 cases. Journal of Orthopaedic Trauma. 1995;**9**:171–176

[22] Manoli AD, Weber TG.Fasciotomy of the foot: An anatomical study with special reference to release of the calcaneal compartment. Foot & Ankle. 1990;**10**(5):267–275

[23] Myerson M, Manoli A. Compartment syndromes of the foot after calcaneal fractures. Clinical Orthopaedics and Related Research. 1993;**290**:142–150

[24] Koval KJ, Sanders R. The radiologic evaluation of calcaneal fractures. Clinical Orthopaedics and Related Research. 1993;**290**:41–46

[25] Davis D, Seaman TJ, Newton EJ. Calcaneus Fractures. [Updated 2023 Jul 31]. In: StatPearls [Internet]. Treasure Island (FL): StatPearls Publishing; 2025 Jan. In: StatPearls. Treasure Island (FL): StatPearls Publishing; 2023

[26] Er A, Murphy A. Broden's View. Radiopaedia.org, Radiology Reference Article. Published Jan 20, 2022. [Accessed: 2025-August-7]

[27] Broden B. Roentgen Examination of the Subtaloid Joint in Fractures of the Calcaneus. Acta Radiologica. 1949;**31**:85–91

[28] Kwon DG, Chung CY, Lee KM, Kim TW, Sung KH, Kim DH, et al. Revisit of Broden's view for intraarticular calcaneal fracture. Clinics in Orthopedic Surgery. 2012;**4**:221–226

[29] Prasartritha T, Sethavanitch C. Three-dimensional and two-dimensional computerized tomographic demonstration of calcaneus fractures. Foot & Ankle International. 2004;**25**:262–273

[30] Janzen DL, Connell DG, Munk PL, et al. Intraarticular fractures of the calcaneus: Value of CT findings in determining prognosis. American Journal of Roentgenology. 1992;**158**:1271–1274

[31] Brenner P, Rammelt S, Gavlik JM, Zwipp H. Early soft tissue coverage after complex foot trauma. World Journal of Surgery. 2001;**25**:603–609

[32] Baumgaertel FR, Gotzen L. Two stage operative treatment of comminuted os calcis fractures: Primary indirect reduction with medial external fixation and delayed lateral plate fixation. Clinical Orthopaedics and Related Research. 1993;**290**: 132–141

[33] Bezes H, Massart P, Delvaux D, et al. The operative treatment of intraarticular calcaneal fractures: Indications, technique, and results in 257 cases. Clinical Orthopaedics and Related Research. 1993;**290**: 55–59

[34] Tornetta P. 3rd. The Essex-Lopresti reduction for calcaneal fractures revisited. Journal of Orthopaedic Trauma. 1998;**12**: 469–473

[35] Zwipp H, Tscherne H, Thermann H, et al. Osteosynthesis of displaced intra-articular fractures of the calcaneus: Results in 123 cases. Clinical Orthopaedics and Related Research. 1993;**290**:76–86

[36] Buckley R, Tough S, McCormack R. Operative compared with nonoperative treatment of displaced intra-articular fractures: A prospective, randomized, controlled multicenter trial. The Journal of Bone and Joint Surgery-American Volume. 2002;**84**:1733–1744

[37] Randle JA, Kreder HJ, Stephen D, et al. Should calcaneal fractures be treated surgically? Clinical Orthopaedics and Related Research. 2000;**377**:217–227

[38] Sharr PJ, Mangupli MM, Winson IG, Buckley RE. Current management options for displaced intra-articular calcaneal fractures: Nonoperative, ORIF, minimally invasive reduction and fixation or primary ORIF and subtalar arthrodesis. A contemporary review. Foot and Ankle Surgery. 2016;**22**:1–8

[39] Rammelt S, Sangeorzan BJ, Swords MP. Calcaneal fractures – Should we or should we not operate? Indian Journal of Orthopaedics. 2018;**52**:220–230. DOI: 10.4103/ortho.IJOrtho_555_17

[40] Rammelt S, Amlang M, Barthel S, Gavlik JM, Zwipp H. Percutaneous treatment of less severe intra-articular calcaneal fractures. Clinical Orthopaedics and Related Research. 2010;**468**:983–990

[41] Tornetta P. 3rd. Percutaneous treatment of calcaneal fractures. Clinical Orthopaedics and Related Research. 2000;**375**:91–96

[42] Gavlik JM, Rammelt S, Zwipp H. Percutaneous, arthroscopically assisted osteosynthesis of calcaneus fractures. Archives of Orthopaedic and Trauma Surgery. 2002;**122**:424–428

[43] Woon CY, Chong KW, Yeo W, Yeo NE, Wong MK. Subtalar arthroscopy and fluoroscopy in percutaneous fixation of intra-articular calcaneal fractures: The best of both worlds. The Journal of Trauma. 2011;**71**:917–925

[44] Stulik J, Stehlik J, Rysavy M, Wozniak A. Minimally-invasive treatment of intraarticular fractures of the calcaneum. The Journal of Bone and Joint Surgery. British Volume. 2006;**88**:1634–1641

[45] Magnan B, Bortolazzi R, Marangon A, Marino M, Dall'Oca C, Bartolozzi P, et al. External fixation for displaced intra-articular fractures of the calcaneum. The Journal of Bone and Joint Surgery. British Volume. 2006;**88**:1474–1479

[46] Smith M, Medlock G, Johnstone AJ. Percutaneous screw fixation of unstable ankle fractures in patients with poor soft tissues and significant co-morbidities. Foot and Ankle Surgery: Official Journal of the European Society of Foot and Ankle Surgeons. 2017;**23**:16–20. DOI: 10.1016/j.fas.2015.11.008

[47] Farrell BM, Lin CA, Moon CN. Temporising external fixation of calcaneus fractures prior to definitive plate fixation: A case series. Injury. 2015;**46**:S19–S22. DOI: 10.1016/s0020-1383(15)30006-1

[48] Tennent TD, Calder PR, Salisbury RD, Allen PW, Eastwood DM. The operative management of displaced intra-articular fractures of the calcaneum: A two-centre study using a defined protocol. Injury. 2001;**32**: 491–496

[49] Thordarson DB, Krieger LE. Operative versus nonoperative treatment of intra-articular fractures of the calcaneus: A prospective, randomized trial. Foot & Ankle International. 1996;**17** (1):2–9

[50] Freeman BJ, Duff S, Allen PE, Nicholson HD, Atkins RM. The extended lateral approach to the hindfoot: Anatomical basis and surgical implications. The Journal of Bone and Joint Surgery. British Volume. 1998;**80**:139–142

[51] Gould N. Lateral approach to the os calcis. Foot & Ankle. 1984;**4**:218–220

[52] Ishikawa K, Kyutoku S, Takeuchi E. Free lateral calcaneal flap. Annals of Plastic Surgery. 1993;**30**: 167–170

[53] Hsu AR, Anderson RB, Cohen BE. Advances in surgical management of intra-articular calcaneus fractures. Journal of the American Academy of Orthopaedic Surgeons. 2015;**23**:399–407

[54] Nosewicz TL, Knupp M, Barg A, et al. Mini-open sinus tarsi approach for fixation of displaced intra-articular calcaneal fractures: A prospective study. Journal of Orthopaedic Trauma. 2012;**26**:638–644

[55] Schepers T. The sinus tarsi approach in displaced intra-articular calcaneal fractures: A systematic review. International Orthopaedics. 2011;**35**:697–703

[56] Ma D, Huang L, Liu B, Liu Z, Xu X, Liu J, et al. Efficacy of Sinus tarsal approach compared with conventional L-shaped lateral approach in the treatment of calcaneal fractures: A meta-analysis. Frontiers in Surgery. 2021;**15**:7

[57] Park Y, Cho WT, Lee M, Lee J, Seo YW. Learning curve of a novice foot and ankle surgeon in minimally invasive calcaneal fracture surgery via the sinus tarsi approach. Scientific Reports. 2025;**15**:27936. DOI: 10.1038/s41598-025-13338-z

[58] Allegra PR, Rivera S, Desai SS, Aiyer A, Kaplan J, Gross CE. Intra-articular calcaneus fractures: Current concepts review. Foot & Ankle Orthopaedics. 2020;**5**:247301142092733

[59] Kline AJ, Anderson RB, Davis WH, et al. Minimally invasive technique versus extensile lateral approach for intra-articular calcaneal fractures. Foot & Ankle International. 2013;**34**:773–780

[60] Burdeaux BD. Fractures of the Calcaneus: Open reduction and internal fixation from the medial side, a 21-year prospective study. Foot & Ankle International. 1997;**18**:685–692

[61] Burdeaux BD. Reduction of calcaneal fractures by the McReynolds medial approach technique and its experimental basis. Clinical Orthopaedics and Related Research. 1983;**177**:87–103

[62] Sivakumar BS, Wong P, Dick CG, Steer RA, Tetsworth K. Arthroscopic reduction and percutaneous fixation of selected calcaneus fractures: Surgical technique and early results. Journal of Orthopaedic Trauma. 2014;**28**:569–576

[63] Gavlik JM, Rammelt S, Zwipp H. The use of subtalar arthroscopy in open reduction and internal fixation of intra-articular calcaneal fractures. Injury. 2002;**33**:63–71. DOI: 10.1016/S0020-1383(01)00077-8

[64] Longino D, Buckley RE. Bone graft in the operative treatment of displaced intra-articular calcaneal fractures: Is it helpful? Journal of Orthopaedic Trauma. 2001;**15**:280–286

[65] Geel CW, Flemister AS. Standardized treatment of intra-articular calcaneal fractures using an oblique lateral incision and no bone graft. The Journal of Trauma: Injury, Infection, and Critical Care. 2001;**50**:1083–1089

[66] Sykes M, Kisson E, Reichert I, Rose V, Ahluwalia R. Infected open calcaneal fractures – A delayed reconstruction technique using calcium sulphate and hydroxyapatite antibiotic elucidating void filler. J Clin Orthop Trauma. 2020;**11**(3):462–466. DOI: 10.1016/j.jcot.2020.03.017

[67] Illert T, Rammelt S, Drewes T, Grass R, Zwipp H. Stability of locking and non-locking plates in an osteoporotic calcaneal fracture model. Foot & Ankle International. 2011;**32**:307–313

[68] Chen K, Zhang H, Wang G, Cheng Y, Qian Z, Yang H. Comparison of nonlocking plates and locking plates for intra-articular calcaneal fractures. Foot & Ankle International. 2014;**35**: 1298–1302. DOI: 10.1177/1071100714547520

[69] Dingemans SA, Sintenie FW, de Jong VM, Luitse JS, Schepers T. Fixation methods for calcaneus fractures: A systematic review of biomechanical studies using cadaver specimens. The Journal of Foot and Ankle Surgery. 2018;**57**:116–122. DOI: 10.1053/j.jfas.2017.05.042

[70] Csizy M, Buckley R, Tough S, Leighton R, Smith J, McCormack R, et al. Displaced intra-articular calcaneal fractures: Variables predicting late subtalar fusion. Journal of Orthopaedic Trauma. 2003;**17**: 106–112

[71] Schepers T. The primary arthrodesis for severely comminuted intra-articular fractures of the calcaneus: A systematic review. Foot and Ankle Surgery. 2012;**18**:84–88

[72] Buckley R, Leighton R, Sanders D, Poon J, Coles CP, Stephen D, et al. Open reduction and internal fixation compared with ORIF and primary

subtalar arthrodesis for treatment of Sanders type IV calcaneal fractures: A randomized multicenter trial. Journal of Orthopaedic Trauma. 2014;**28**: 577–583. DOI: 10.1097/BOT.0000000000000191

[73] Fadle AA, Fadle MA, Elgeidy A, Fadle SA. Extensible lateral approach versus sinus tarsi approach for Sanders II–III displaced intra-articular calcaneal fractures. Journal of Orthopaedic Surgery and Research. 2025;**20**:83. DOI: 10.1186/s13018-024-05345-z

[74] de Boer AS, van Lieshout EMM, Moolenbroek G, den Hartog D, Verhofstad MHJ. The effect of time to postoperative weight-bearing on outcomes in displaced intra-articular calcaneal fractures: Systematic review and pooled analysis. Injury. 2018;**49**:743–752. DOI: 10.1016/j.injury.2018.02.017

[75] Verstappen C, Sosef N, van der Vliet QMJ, van Lieshout EMM, Hietbrink F, Houwert RM, et al. The role of early weight bearing in the aftertreatment of unilateral displaced intra-articular calcaneal fractures: Systematic review and pooled analysis. Journal of Orthopaedics and Traumatology. 2025;**26**:17. DOI: 10.1186/s10195-025-00863

[76] Verstappen C, Kalmet PHS, Maduro CV, VAN Vugt R, Sintenie JB, VAN DER Veen A, Edwards MJR, Poeze M, Hermans E, Driessen mls. patient-reported outcomes after permissive weight bearing in surgically treated trauma patients with displaced intra-articular calcaneal fractures: a multicentre, retrospective cohort study. J Rehabil Med Clin Commun. 2025;**8**:42747. DOI: 10.2340/jrm-cc.v8.42747

[77] Chongmuenwai A, Thitirangsi T. Outcomes of Early Weight Bearing in Displaced Intra-articular Calcaneus Fractures Treated with Screws-Only Fixation Technique. JOIO. 2023;**57**: 461–465. DOI: 10.1007/s43465-023-00823-8

[78] Stephenson JR. Treatment of displaced intra-articular fractures of the calcaneus using medial and lateral approaches, internal fixation, and early motion. The Journal of Bone & Joint Surgery. 1987;**69**:115–130

[79] Carr JB, Hansen ST, Benirschke SK. Subtalar distraction bone block fusion for late complications of os calcis fractures. Foot & Ankle. 1988;**9**:81–86

[80] Romash MM. Reconstructive osteotomy of the calcaneus with subtalar arthrodesis for malunited calcaneal fractures. Clinical Orthopaedics and Related Research. 1993;**290**:157–167

[81] Rammelt S, Zwipp H. Corrective arthrodeses and osteotomies for post-traumatic hindfoot malalignment: Indications, techniques, results. International Orthopaedics. 2013;**37**:1707–1717. DOI: 10.1007/s00264-013-2021-3

Section 3

Complex and Challenging Fracture Scenarios

Chapter 6

Fracture Nonunion

Khalil Nasrallah, Fadi Abboud, Einal Bathish and Haim Shtarker

Abstract

Fracture nonunion remains a considerable challenge in orthopedic trauma, particularly in the tibia and femur, where the mechanical environment, soft-tissue compromise, and host factors converge. This chapter synthesizes current concepts spanning definition, classification, and pathophysiology and translates them into pragmatic diagnostic and therapeutic algorithms for orthopedic surgeons. This chapter also outlines risk stratification across mechanical instability, biological insufficiency, and systemic determinants, and provides a stepwise approach to clinical, radiographic, and adjunct investigations to differentiate delayed union from nonunion and to screen for occult infection. Surgical strategies are presented with an emphasis on contemporary evidence comparing exchange intramedullary nailing with augmentative plating over a retained nail; for femoral shaft nonunion, augmentative plating with autologous graft is highlighted as a preferred option given faster union and fewer complications, while both approaches remain effective in the tibia with selection tailored to anatomy, alignment, and biology. The role of bone grafting (iliac crest and RIA harvests), scaffold extenders, and bone marrow aspirate concentrate is critically appraised, alongside biophysical adjuncts such as pulsed electromagnetic fields and low-intensity pulsed ultrasound. Complex scenarios, including infected nonunion, segmental defects, and deformity, are addressed using staged debridement, antibiotic strategies, Masquelet-induced membrane reconstruction, bone transport, and vascularized grafts.

Keywords: fracture nonunion, tibial nonunion, femoral nonunion, exchange nailing, augmentative plating, bone grafting, pulsed electromagnetic fields, low-intensity pulsed ultrasound, infected nonunion, Masquelet technique

1. Introduction

Fracture nonunion is considered a challenging complication in orthopedic trauma, often resulting in prolonged patient morbidity and substantial healthcare costs. Despite advancements in surgical techniques and technology, the incidence of long bone fracture nonunion has remained significant; roughly 5%–10% of all fractures (10%–15% of surgically managed fractures) fail to unite within expected timeframes [1, 2]. Tibial shaft fractures, in particular, have the highest nonunion rates among long bones (the reported incidence ranges from around 1% in low-risk cases up to 19% in severe cases), while the nonunion rate of femoral fractures is between 10% and 12%, depending on injury severity [1]. These statistics underscore the tibia and femur as frequent sites of nonunion, often due to the tibia's subcutaneous location and tenuous blood supply, as well as the high-energy mechanisms associated with tibial and femoral fractures.

Nonunions impose a heavy burden on both patients and the healthcare system. They lead to prolonged disability, repeated surgeries, and psychosocial distress. Economically, the cost of treating a nonunion is dramatically higher than that of an uncomplicated fracture. One analysis showed that the average total cost of care for patients with a nonunion was nearly three times higher than for patients whose fractures healed normally ($102,000 vs. $35,000 in one study) [1]. In the United States, an open tibia fracture nonunion incurs a median cost of $25,000, roughly double that of a similar fracture that achieves union [2]. Beyond direct costs, nonunion patients experience extended loss of work income (often between 6 and 12 months or more of work absence) and higher utilization of healthcare resources, including increased use of analgesics (opioids/nonsteroidal anti-inflammatory drugs [NSAIDs]) for chronic pain.

The impact on patient quality of life is profound. Persistently unhealed fractures cause chronic pain, functional limitations, and psychological distress [2]. Studies have found that patients with tibial or femoral nonunion report significantly worse physical and mental health scores than those who healed normally, with higher rates of depression, reliance on assistive devices, and earlier retirement due to disability [1]. These considerations highlight that fracture nonunion is not only an orthopedic problem confined to bone healing but a complex condition affecting the whole patient [3]. In light of this, it is crucial that the orthopedic surgeon understands that nonunion is rarely a simple or single-factor process but rather a complex, multifaceted condition and that evidence-based tools are available to promote bone healing.

2. Definition and classification

Definition: Fracture nonunion has long been difficult to define with precision, as it represents a failure of normal healing rather than a distinct time-bound event. Traditionally, the U.S. Food and Drug Administration (FDA) definition (circa 1998) is cited: a nonunion is "established" by nine months post-fracture with no visible progressive healing for at least three consecutive months [1, 2]. In clinical practice, many surgeons diagnose and treat a "nonunion" earlier, often around six months post-fracture, if there are no signs of healing progress on serial radiographs and the clinical picture suggests the fracture will not heal without intervention [1]. The Danish Orthopedic Trauma Society has proposed a more pragmatic definition: "a fracture that will not heal without further intervention." This highlights that the essence of nonunion is the biological inability to heal spontaneously, rather than an absolute time frame. However, this pragmatic definition still requires the clinician to judge when healing has ceased. In practice, a combination of chronological and clinical criteria is used: if a fracture shows no radiographic bridging and clinically persistent pain or instability by around six months (sooner in the absence of any healing progress), it is generally considered a nonunion, especially if serial X-rays over a two- to three-month period show no callus progression and maturation. It is important to distinguish a true nonunion from a "delayed union," which implies slow healing that may still complete given more time; typically, delayed union is suspected by three to six months when healing is not on track [2].

Despite attempts at consensus, there is no single universally accepted definition of nonunion that captures both the time element and the biological aspect [2]. Various scoring systems (e.g., the Radiographic Union Scale for Tibial fractures (RUST)) and definitions (e.g., FDA, Medicare, etc.) exist, which can complicate diagnosis and research inclusion criteria.

Classification: Once a nonunion is identified, classification helps guide treatment and communicate the underlying pathology. The most commonly used classification is based on the radiographic appearance and inferred biology of the nonunion, as described by Weber and Cech [4]. This scheme broadly divides nonunions into three categories [4]:

- Hypertrophic (Hypervascular) nonunion: Abundant callus formation is seen on X-ray, but the fracture fails to bridge. This "elephant foot" or hypertrophic callus indicates that the biology (blood supply, osteogenesis) is robust; the primary problem is usually mechanical instability. In hypertrophic nonunions, the body is producing callus in response to motion, but the excessive interfragmentary movement prevents consolidation. These are viable nonunions with a "favorable biological response" but inadequate stability [4].

- Atrophic (Avascular) nonunion: Minimal or no callus is visible. The fracture ends may be sclerotic or atrophic ("pencil tip" appearance) with a gap. This reflects an unfavorable biological environment and a poor healing response, often due to insufficient blood supply, extensive cortical devitalization, or large bone loss. Atrophic nonunions are nonviable; the biology is quiescent and needs enhancement in addition to stability. These cases often require aggressive measures to stimulate healing, such as debridement of sclerotic bone and the addition of grafts or growth factors [4].

- Oligotrophic nonunion: An intermediate category characterized by little to moderate callus that does not progress to union. It is sometimes considered a subset of viable nonunion, where there is some biological activity, but perhaps not in the optimal location or amount to achieve union. Oligotrophic nonunions often result from fracture fragments that are not apposed (distraction or a gap) or from inadequate reduction, which leads to fibrous tissue rather than mineralized callus bridging the gap. They "bridge the gap" between hypertrophic and atrophic cases in terms of biology; the healing response is present but not effective enough [4].

Another crucial practical classification distinction is between septic and aseptic nonunion. An aseptic nonunion has no evidence of infection, whereas a septic (infected) nonunion indicates that the fracture site is harboring an infection (chronic osteomyelitis), which can inhibit healing. This distinction is critical because the presence of infection radically alters the treatment approach, requiring debridement, antibiotics, and often staged reconstruction. Any nonunion classification system must account for infection status. For example, the Cierny–Mader classification, originally developed for osteomyelitis, is sometimes applied to infected nonunions, taking into account the host's physiological status and the local bony involvement (medullary, superficial, segmental, etc.).

Host Factors Classification: There have also been attempts to classify nonunions by host and injury factors. One such approach is the "Nonunion Risk Score" or Calori classification, which assigns points for risk factors (like smoking, diabetes, soft tissue damage, etc.) to stratify the difficulty of healing. While not a formal part of nonunion nomenclature, considering host factors is important; for instance, the Nonunion Scoring System (NUSS) helps predict which fractures are at high risk for nonunion and might benefit from early intervention [2].

It should be noted that traditional radiographic classifications have limitations. They are based on static X-ray appearances and may not capture issues like infection or systemic factors. Mills et al. [5] emphasized that radiographic classification alone can be misleading and should be used in conjunction with a thorough clinical and etiological assessment. In Mills' series of 100 nonunions, only 31% had a single identifiable cause; the majority (69%) had two or more contributing factors. Moreover, 5% of ostensibly "aseptic" nonunions in that series turned out to have unexpected infections on culture. These findings highlight that nonunions are often multifactorial – a combination of mechanical, biological, and patient factors – and that careful evaluation, including microbiology, is necessary rather than relying solely on the X-ray appearance [5].

3. Pathophysiology

Why do fractures go on to nonunion? The pathophysiology of nonunion can be understood as a failure in one (or more) of the fundamental requirements for bone healing. The "Diamond Concept" of fracture healing describes four essential components: (1) a mechanically stable environment, (2) osteogenic cells, (3) an osteoconductive scaffold, and (4) osteoinductive growth factors [6]. If any of these components is insufficient, the fracture may not heal. Broadly, the causes of nonunion are often categorized into mechanical factors, biological factors, infectious factors, and host (systemic) factors [5]. These roughly correspond to problems with stability, local biology (including blood supply), the presence of infection, and patient-related issues, respectively.

- Mechanical pathophysiology: Bone healing is highly sensitive to the mechanical environment. According to Perren's strain theory, if interfragmentary strain (the change in gap length under loading, divided by gap length) exceeds approximately 2%, bony bridging is inhibited; high strain leads to fibrous tissue or cartilage instead of bone [5]. In an adequately stabilized fracture, interfragmentary strain drops as callus forms. However, if a fracture has inadequate stabilization (e.g., insufficient fixation rigidity or an excessive gap), the motion at the fracture site remains too great for mineralized bone to form. Instead, the fracture ends may develop abundant callus that never fully bridges (resulting in a hypertrophic nonunion), or in cases of a large gap, even callus formation is thwarted and a fibrovascular nonunion forms. A classical example is a comminuted fracture fixed with a plate that is too small or with insufficient fixation points, leading to micromotion that stimulates callus but not union. Large fracture gaps are particularly problematic: Experimental data show that even with rigid fixation, a critical size gap can fail to heal because the initial bridging tissue cannot span the distance [5].

- Biological pathophysiology: The flip side is an environment where stability might be adequate, but the biology is compromised. Bone healing requires a viable osteogenic response, an adequate population of progenitor cells that can form bone, and a supportive blood supply to nurture those cells. If the fracture fragments are devascularized, the bone ends may simply not generate callus. Early vascularity is crucial; insufficient revascularization of the fracture site predisposes it to an atrophic nonunion [5]. Causes of biological failure include poor local blood supply, extensive bone loss (no scaffold or cells present in the gap), or extinction of cellular activity due to factors like radiation, infection, or excessive periosteal injury [7]. The fracture ends can become "inert," effectively walled off by sclerotic bone or scar tissue. The radiographic atrophic appearance correlates with this scenario. Additionally, certain medications (e.g., chronic high-dose steroids or prolonged use of NSAIDs, which interfere with inflammation and bone formation) can suppress the biological healing response. If biology is the limiting factor, simply adding stability (e.g., re-fixation) without addressing the biological deficit (through bone grafting or stimulatory factors) may not succeed. This is why atrophic nonunions usually require both debridement of poorly vascular bone and the addition of autograft or other adjuncts to reinitiate healing.

- Infection: The presence of infection profoundly alters the healing environment. Osteomyelitis at the fracture site leads to persistent inflammation, osteolysis, and often instability as hardware loosens in infected tissue [5]. Bacteria form biofilms on implants and devitalized bone, interfering with osteogenesis. Even if a fracture was initially adequately stabilized, an indolent infection can cause what would otherwise be a healthy callus to halt and resorb. Infected nonunions often have a mix of mechanical and biological issues: Infection induces bone resorption and may create a gap, while the body's attempt to clear the infection can divert resources away from regenerative processes. The result is often a recalcitrant nonunion with sequestra (dead bone) and drainage. Notably, infection can present subtly; for example, a fracture that simply fails to heal (so-called "occult infection" nonunion) without obvious signs of infection. In one series, all patients who had been previously treated for infection and then believed to be aseptic were found to have positive cultures at revision, indicating that any history of infection should raise suspicion in a nonunion [5]. Given the high stakes, routine deep cultures are recommended in nonunion surgery to rule out infection, even in cases that appear aseptic. Infection pathophysiology in nonunion mandates a two-front battle: Eradication of bacteria and promotion of bone healing.

- Systemic/Host factors: The patient's overall health and habits critically influence bone healing. Smoking is one of the most well-documented risk factors for delayed healing and nonunion; nicotine and other tobacco metabolites cause vasoconstriction and impair osteoblast function, roughly doubling the risk of nonunion in long bone fractures. Studies consider heavy smoking (e.g., > 1 pack/day or ≥ 10 cigarettes/day) a significant risk factor [8]. Diabetes mellitus, especially if poorly controlled, impairs wound and bone healing by reducing cellular function and blood flow. Other chronic diseases, such as renal failure or anemia, can compromise healing as well. Nutritional status (e.g., vitamin D levels, protein intake) matters: malnutrition or deficiencies can reduce the substrate needed for bone repair. Certain medications, like chronic steroids (which inhibit osteoblasts and prolong inflammation) or NSAIDs (which, when used for prolonged periods early in fracture healing, have been shown in animal models to impair callus formation), can predispose to nonunion [5]. Age is a factor too; older patients heal more slowly due to lower osteogenic cell populations and comorbidities. Additionally, the concept of "biological aging" of a fracture – a long delay in intervention (fracture fragments left with motion for many months) – can lead to a state where the healing responses have burned out and scar tissue has filled the gap, making later healing attempts more difficult. Host immune status is important in infected cases; immunosuppressed or ill patients may not contain infection or mount a healing response well. In summary, systemic factors such as smoking, diabetes, vascular disease, alcoholism, and advanced age are recognized contributors to nonunion risk [2]. Often, these act in concert with local factors, for example, a smoker with a badly comminuted open tibia has a compounded risk.

In summary, the pathogenesis of tibial and femoral nonunions can be traced to failures in mechanics (too much or too little stability) and/or biology (inadequate blood supply or cells), often compounded by infection or systemic issues. A hypertrophic nonunion indicates that biology is intact but stability was insufficient; an atrophic nonunion indicates biological failure (and often also a mechanical issue, such as a gap or poor vascularity). These are two ends of a spectrum. The surgeon must interpret the nonunion's appearance and history to determine the dominant causes. Understanding these mechanisms underpins the rational selection of treatments. For example, a purely hypertrophic nonunion might heal with improved stabilization alone, whereas an atrophic nonunion will require a biological boost (graft or growth factors) in addition to stabilization. The "Diamond" concept reminds us that bone healing is achieved when stability, cells, scaffold, and signals are all present; the pathophysiology of nonunion lies in the absence of one or more of these critical factors.

4. Nonoperative management of nonunion

By the time a fracture meets the criteria for nonunion, surgical intervention is the definitive treatment in the vast majority of cases, especially for tibial and femoral shaft nonunions. These are weight-bearing bones where a stable union is critical for function; thus, leaving them ununited is usually not acceptable long-term. That said, there are some limited scenarios and adjunct measures in which nonoperative or minimally invasive strategies might be employed, either in an attempt to avoid surgery or as a temporizing measure. It should be emphasized that nonoperative approaches are generally more successful in delayed unions or very early nonunions, as opposed to established, refractory nonunions. Once a nonunion is well-established (especially if the fragments are sclerotic or there is significant deformity), purely non-surgical management has a low likelihood of success.

Prolonged immobilization and functional bracing: The simplest nonoperative management involves giving the fracture more time with continued immobilization (cast or bracing) and protected weight-bearing. Historically, before modern surgical methods, some fractures that had not united after several months were treated with extended casting or functional braces, allowing partial weight-bearing to stimulate healing (Wolff's law states that mechanical stimulation encourages bone formation). For instance, Sarmiento's functional brace for tibial fractures can sometimes help a slowly healing tibia achieve union by allowing controlled motion and weight-bearing in a brace. In modern practice, if a fracture shows some progress but is slow (delayed union), one might continue immobilization beyond the typical timeframe rather than operate immediately. However, simply keeping a truly stagnant fracture in a cast indefinitely is usually futile. There are cases, often anecdotal, of very late unions (e.g., a fracture finally unites after 18 months), but relying on that is not advisable if no progress is evident by six to nine months. An exception might be in a patient who is non-ambulatory or has low demand; for example, in a very elderly patient with minimal pain, one might treat a fibrous nonunion conservatively if the function is acceptable.

Dynamization of existing fixation: This is a minimally invasive "semi-operative" strategy particularly applicable to fractures treated with intramedullary nails. Nail dynamization involves removing one or more locking screws from the nail (typically the static interlocking screw that prevents collapse) to allow the fracture ends to come closer and introduce some axial micromotion. The rationale is that controlled compression and slight motion can stimulate callus formation if the fracture was too rigid or if there was a small gap preventing contact. Dynamization is usually attempted in around three to four months if a nailed fracture shows delayed healing but some callus presence. In the context of nonunion, dynamization is more likely to help in a hypertrophic or oligotrophic scenario where biology is present but perhaps the fracture ends are held apart or too rigidly fixed. It is generally not useful for atrophic nonunions (where biology is absent) or when there is a large gap. Additionally, dynamization only helps if the nail was initially statically locked; if the fracture was already dynamized or if all screws are already out (as in an unlocked nail), then this option is not available. Historical data on nail dynamization success are mixed. Older series reported union achieved in roughly 50%–70% of cases when dynamization was done for delayed union [9]. A recent review notes that success rates for nail dynamization in established tibial/femoral shaft nonunions are on the order of 55%–65% [10], meaning nearly half of cases will still require further surgery. Therefore, dynamization is generally considered in the earlier phase of a developing nonunion (delayed union) as a first step, but if significant healing does not occur in the next two to three months post-dynamization, more invasive measures (such as exchange nailing) are indicated [10]. One must also ensure that dynamization will actually transmit load across the fracture. For example, if a fracture has a large gap or the nail has a bend, simply removing screws may not lead to compression, and in such cases, dynamization could even create too much instability. Additionally, there is a risk: if the fracture still does not heal, removing screws can lead to hardware failure (excessive motion causing nail breakage or deformity) [9].

External bone stimulation: Two primary modalities exist – pulsed electromagnetic field (PEMF) stimulation and low-intensity pulsed ultrasound (LIPUS). These modalities are noninvasive treatments applied externally to the limb that aim to stimulate bone healing through biophysical signals. They are among the few FDA-approved nonoperative treatments specifically indicated for aiding nonunion healing.

- PEMF: The patient uses coils or a device that emits electromagnetic fields around the nonunion site for several hours a day. Clinical evidence has shown that PEMF can induce healing in a significant proportion of nonunions, with reported success rates ranging from 73% to 85% in various series. In practice, PEMF is often prescribed for patients who are not good surgical candidates or who refuse surgery. It can also be used as an adjunct to surgery. We often request a PEMF device for a patient with a recalcitrant tibial nonunion as a supplement to surgical revision, especially if the biology is poor [11].

- LIPUS: This is an ultrasound device (e.g., Exogen) applied daily that delivers low-intensity ultrasound waves to the fracture. LIPUS has been shown in some studies to accelerate the healing of fresh fractures and some nonunions by promoting callus formation and angiogenesis [12]. It has the advantage of being easy to use at home for 20 minutes daily. Like PEMF, it is often employed in scenarios where surgery is being delayed or avoided. For instance, if a patient's fracture shows minimal healing at four months, adding LIPUS might convert it to union by six to seven months, obviating surgery. Some meta-analyses suggest that LIPUS can significantly shorten the time to union in nonunions/ delayed unions [12]. It is considered a safe, cost-effective modality with essentially no systemic risks, though patient compliance is needed.

It is important to note that nonoperative adjuncts like bone stimulators are more likely to succeed in aiding a healing response that is slow, as in delayed nonunion, rather than creating one from nothing. For example, a hypertrophic tibial nonunion with lots of callus might benefit from ultrasound or PEMF to "push it over the edge." In contrast, a totally atrophic, mobile nonunion with a big gap is unlikely to unite with a stimulator alone. Nonetheless, in certain patients (e.g., those who cannot undergo surgery due to medical issues), a course of PEMF or LIPUS is worth trying, as it may induce enough bone formation to achieve union or at least a pain-free fibrous union.

Pharmacological adjuncts: There is ongoing research into systemic therapies that might promote fracture healing. One example is teriparatide (recombinant PTH 1–34), an anabolic osteoporosis drug that has shown some promise in case reports for enhancing difficult fracture healing. While not standard, some surgeons have used off-label teriparatide daily injections for a few months to encourage callus formation in a delayed union. Results are anecdotal but biologically plausible, as PTH can stimulate osteoblasts [13]. Similarly, optimizing the patient's biology with nutritional supplementation (vitamin D, calcium, protein) is sensible if deficiencies are found. Good endocrinological health (thyroid, parathyroid, etc., in balance) is important – rarely, an undiagnosed metabolic bone disorder could be contributing, so in refractory cases, checking for osteoporosis or other metabolic issues can be considered.

In summary, nonoperative management of nonunion is limited. Extended immobilization, functional bracing, and delaying surgery might be attempted in the hope of late union, but success is far from guaranteed. Biophysical stimulation (PEMF, LIPUS) can be valuable adjunct therapies, having shown the ability to induce union in a substantial fraction of cases without surgical intervention. For certain patients, these modalities offer a chance to avoid another operation. Nail dynamization is a minor intervention that can help some delayed unions consolidate without a full reoperation, particularly in well-aligned fractures lacking only compression. Ultimately, if these measures do not yield clear signs of healing within a couple of months, the surgeon should proceed to operative management rather than prolong the patient's disability. Keeping the patient engaged in weight-bearing (when safe) and physical therapy for joint motion is also important during any nonoperative trial, because maintaining limb function will aid recovery once union is achieved (either spontaneously or after later surgery).

5. Surgical treatment strategies

When nonoperative measures are insufficient or inappropriate, surgical intervention is required to achieve union. Indeed, for most tibial and femoral nonunions, surgery is the definitive solution. The goals of surgery in a nonunion are twofold: (1) provide a stable mechanical environment (usually by internal or external fixation) and (2) enhance the biological environment (often by debridement of fibrous tissue and nonviable bone, and addition of bone graft or other osteogenic material) [10]. These principles apply broadly, but the optimal surgical strategy can differ between the tibia and femur due to anatomical and biomechanical considerations. Furthermore, the strategy depends on the type of nonunion (hypertrophic vs. atrophic) and whether infection is present. This section will focus on aseptic diaphyseal nonunions of the tibia and femur, discussing the typical surgical options and the evidence behind them – notably the contemporary debate of exchange intramedullary nailing versus augmentative plating for nonunions after initial intramedullary nailing.

5.1 Tibial nonunion

Initial considerations: The tibial shaft is commonly stabilized with an intramedullary nail for acute fractures. Thus, many tibial nonunions present as an unhealed fracture with a nail in place. Others may occur after plate fixation or external fixation. Deciding on the surgical approach involves analyzing why the tibia did not heal: Was it primarily a stability issue (suggesting the need for improved fixation), a biology issue (suggesting the need for bone grafting), or both? Key factors in tibial nonunion management include alignment (any malalignment should be corrected during surgery), the condition of the soft tissues (sometimes residual wounds or the need for flap coverage), and the presence of any infection. Assuming an aseptic tibial nonunion, the classic options are Exchange reamed nailing, augmentative plate fixation (with or without removing the nail), and in some cases, external fixation if needed (particularly for very complex cases or if multiple attempts have failed).

Exchange nailing: This has long been considered the gold standard for aseptic tibial shaft nonunions after a nail [9, 14]. The technique involves removing the current nail, freshening the medullary canal with reamers (usually reaming to a larger diameter, which provides internal bone graft from the reamings and increases endosteal blood flow), and inserting a new, larger-diameter intramedullary nail [10]. Typically, the new nail is 1–2 mm larger in diameter to increase stability ("up-nailing"). Union rates with exchange nailing of the tibia are generally high, reported in the range of 76% to 96% success in various series [14]. These high rates presume good technique, including thorough reaming to remove fibrous tissue, achieving a tight fit of the nail, and locking it appropriately (and sometimes dynamizing it later, if needed). Exchange nailing addresses both mechanics (a stiffer nail and fresh locking screws improve stability) and biology (reaming debris acts as autograft and reaming also works by inducing a new inflammatory response in the canal). Many surgeons also perform cortical bone grafting at the nonunion site during exchange nailing: After reaming and before inserting the new nail, they may take some of the reamed bone material (often collected by the reamer–irrigator–aspirator (RIA) device, if used) and pack it into the fracture gap [15]. Even without deliberate graft packing, the reamings that are forced into the fracture site can have a positive effect (this is sometimes called the "internal bone graft" of exchange nailing). A critical part of exchange nailing is achieving good fracture apposition; if there is a gap, one might consider doing an open exposure to remove interposed fibrous tissue and ensure the bone ends contact. In some cases, especially if the original nonunion had a deformity or misalignment, the surgeon will formally open the nonunion, debride it, correct alignment, and then insert the new nail (this is sometimes called an "opened exchange nailing"). If alignment is acceptable and there is some fibrous tissue, others will perform it closed, letting the reamer clear the tissue.

Augmentative plating ("Plate-over-Nail" technique): This approach has gained popularity in recent years as an alternative to re-nailing. In an augmentative plating procedure, the original nail is typically left in place (if it is well-positioned), and a plate is applied to the fracture site to provide additional stability. The plate is usually a compression or locking plate applied percutaneously or through a limited open approach, spanning the nonunion. The idea is to augment the existing fixation: the nail controls the alignment and takes some load, while the plate adds rotational and bending stiffness, significantly improving overall stability [10]. During this procedure, the nonunion site is often exposed via a small incision to allow for decortication (scraping the bone ends to bleeding bone) and bone grafting (usually autologous cancellous graft from the iliac crest or another source, placed around the nonunion) before the plate is fixed. Essentially, augmentative plating addresses both stability (very rigid due to the nail + plate construct) and biology (by adding bone graft and freshening the bone ends). An advantage of this method is that one does not disturb the intramedullary canal significantly (as opposed to exchange nailing, which involves re-reaming the canal and potential weakening of the bone or risk of a new fracture during nail insertion). Plate-over-nail can be particularly useful if the nonunion has an element of axial malalignment that can be corrected with the plate by shifting one fragment relative to the nail slightly (though large deformities typically require nail removal or osteotomy).

Clinical outcomes for augmentative plating of tibial nonunions have been very encouraging. Several studies report high union rates comparable to or exceeding those of exchange nailing. For instance, in the study by Birjandinejad et al. [16], combined femoral and tibial nonunions were treated with plate-over-nail and achieved union in 100% of femur cases and 84.6% of tibia cases.

However, it is important to select cases properly for augmentative plating. If the original nail is badly malpositioned (e.g., significant malalignment or if the nail is broken), one might not want to keep it; in those cases, exchange nailing or nail removal and plating anew would be chosen. Augmentative plating works best when the nail is in an acceptable position but union did not occur (perhaps due to inadequate stability or biological reasons). By leaving the nail, one maintains alignment and also avoids having to fill the canal after nail removal (which would leave a stress-riser). The plate is encouraged to be placed using the minimally invasive percutaneous osteosynthesis (MIPO) technique, preserving blood supply.

Exchange nailing versus augmentative plating in tibia: For a long time, exchange nailing has been the go-to solution for tibial nonunions post-nailing [10]. However, recently, more surgeons are using plate-over-nail, especially in tricky cases (for example, a tibia that has failed one exchange nailing already or a tibia with a short end-segment that a nail alone struggles to stabilize). The question arises: which is better as a first-line revision for aseptic tibial nonunion after nailing? High-level evidence specifically in tibia is limited; no large randomized trial focusing on tibial nonunions alone has been published to date. There is a shortage of randomized controlled trials (RCTs) and meta-analyses specifically in tibia.

It's worth mentioning that one can also perform "exchange nailing plus augmentative plating" in extreme cases, though that typically means removing the old nail, inserting a new nail, and also adding a plate. That's rarely necessary initially but has been done in recalcitrant cases or in some difficult femur nonunions.

Plating after failed plate fixation: Not all tibial nonunions result from nails. If a tibial fracture was initially plated and progressed to nonunion, the revision options are re-plating (often with a larger, stronger plate and graft), switching to an intramedullary nail (if the fracture pattern allows it), or using external fixation (such as an Ilizarov frame). Re-plating with a compression plate and adding bone graft is a common approach for atrophic tibial nonunions that were initially plated. Switching to a nail can be performed if the alignment is acceptable and the soft tissues can accommodate a nail (for example, if an open wound has healed and there is sufficient bone stock to ream a nail). Classic work by Wiss and Stetson [17] demonstrated the success of intramedullary nailing for tibial nonunions after failed plating. Conversely, compression plating has been used after failures of other methods, including external fixation [10]. Essentially, the surgeon must determine which method will provide the best stability for the specific nonunion configuration.

External fixation: In tibial nonunions with significant bone loss or infection, circular external fixation (Ilizarov or Taylor Spatial Frame) can be used to both stabilize and gradually achieve union (sometimes via bone transport or compression techniques). In aseptic cases with intact bone length, external fixators are less commonly chosen if internal fixation is feasible, because patient comfort and joint motion are generally better with internal fixation. However, if the soft-tissue condition is poor (risk of wound complications from internal hardware) or if multiple surgeries have failed, a period of external fixation can sometimes get a tibia to heal by stimulating callus (mechanical stimulation from the frame can be modulated) and by allowing compression or distraction osteogenesis as needed [10]. For an aseptic tibial nonunion with no bone loss, normally you would not jump to an Ilizarov unless internal methods are contraindicated or have failed.

Bone grafting and adjuncts: Virtually all tibial nonunion surgeries (except perhaps the most hypertrophic ones) include some form of bone graft or bone graft substitute application [18]. For the tibia, autologous cancellous bone graft from the iliac crest is commonly added at the nonunion site, especially if atrophic. The RIA technique can harvest a large volume of bone graft from the femur or tibia, which is a popular method to avoid an extensive iliac crest harvest. This can be done concurrently if one is exchanging a nail (ream extra to collect graft). In augmentative plating, one typically opens the nonunion, resects any scar tissue or sclerotic bone (until the "paprika sign" of punctate bone bleeding is achieved), packs the area with bone graft, and then applies the plate [10]. The combination of decortication and grafting is often termed the classic "Müller's technique" for atrophic nonunions – decortication (opening the bone ends to bleeding bone) and stable fixation with graft yields a high union rate.

Tibial nonunion outcome: With appropriate surgical management, union rates for aseptic tibial nonunions are high, often above 90% after one well-planned intervention [14]. For example, exchange nailing achieves a success rate of 90%, as noted, and augmentative plating yields similarly high results. The time to union after revision is typically in the range of four to six months for plating or nailing, as reported in many series [19]. If the first revision fails, further surgery – sometimes using a different method or adding additional biological enhancements such as bone morphogenetic proteins (BMPs) or cell therapy – can salvage most remaining cases. In summary, for tibial nonunion: Exchange intramedullary nailing has been the workhorse for aseptic tibial shaft nonunions, boasting high union rates (76%–96% in the literature). Augmentative plating (plate-over-nail) is an increasingly popular alternative that provides excellent stability and high union rates, and may lead to faster healing in some cases [16]. The choice of method may depend on the specific scenario; augmentative plating can be especially useful if nail removal is undesirable or if additional stability is needed beyond what a nail can achieve (e.g., distal tibia). Both methods often incorporate bone grafting to maximize success. Good surgical technique – including adequate fixation, alignment, decortication, and infection vigilance – is crucial. In recalcitrant cases or those with bone loss, techniques such as bone transport with external fixation or the Masquelet induced-membrane two-stage grafting come into play [10]. However, for most routine tibial nonunions without infection, a single-stage internal fixation (either exchange nail or nail + plate) with grafting offers an excellent chance of union and return to function.

5.2 Femoral nonunion

Management principles for femoral shaft nonunions are similar to those for the tibia in terms of requiring stability and biology, but the femur has some unique aspects. The femoral shaft is almost always treated primarily with an intramedullary nail (except in certain cases, such as periprosthetic fractures or fractures that are very proximal or distal, requiring plate fixation). Therefore, as with the tibia, a common scenario is a femoral shaft fracture initially treated with a nail that failed to unite. Femoral nonunions can be particularly challenging because the femur experiences high mechanical loads, and patients often expect a pain-free, full weight-bearing function. A nonunion in the femur is very limiting, as patients usually cannot walk without assistive devices or a limp.

Options for aseptic femoral shaft nonunion after nailing: The two main competing strategies are Exchange Nailing versus Augmentative Plating (Plate-over-Nail), analogous to the tibia. Historically, exchange nailing was standard for the femur as well and indeed has a solid success rate reported (often in the 75–95% range) [14]. However, the femur is a larger bone and experiences more torsional stress, and it has been observed that some femoral nonunions (especially when there is a bit of a gap or if the nail is of relatively smaller diameter) might benefit from the added rigidity of a plate.

Exchange nailing (femur): This involves removing the initial nail, reaming the canal larger (often significantly larger, because femoral canals can accommodate large nails), and inserting a new nail with a bigger diameter (and sometimes a different locking configuration if needed). Reaming the femur not only helps insert a larger nail but also promotes a healing response through endosteal bleeding and autografting with reamings. Exchange nailing is classically effective for most femoral shaft nonunions unless specific issues, such as a very distal fracture or a segmental bone defect, are present. In earlier series, initial exchange nailing healed roughly three-quarters of femoral nonunions, with overall union rates approaching or exceeding 90%–100% after additional interventions, especially when a systematic protocol (larger nail, static locking, metabolic optimization, dynamization when needed) was used [14, Swanson et al., 2015]. Exchange nailing in the femur might have a slightly lower first-pass success rate than in the tibia in some older reports, possibly because some femoral nonunions had issues that a nail alone could not fix (such as a large gap requiring bone grafting). In principle, though, a properly performed exchange nailing with up-sizing and possibly static locking (with later dynamization if needed) works for many femoral nonunions.

Augmentative plating (femur): In recent years, augmentative plating of femoral nonunions has been studied extensively, and evidence suggests it may outperform exchange nailing in many cases. The technique is similar: Leave the original nail in place, open the nonunion minimally to clean out fibrous tissue, add bone graft, and apply a strong plate (usually a broad 4.5 mm locking compression plate) bridging the nonunion [20]. By essentially "double plating" the bone (nail inside plus plate outside), the construct becomes extremely stiff, particularly in torsion and bending. The exchange nail construct allows the most rotational motion at the nonunion, which is undesirable for healing. Their conclusion: A robust augmentative plate (4.5 mm) is biomechanically superior to exchange nailing in stabilizing a femoral shaft nonunion. This biomechanical evidence aligns with clinical observations that plating over a nail tends to stop the interfragmentary motion that might be hindering union, especially in cases where a nail alone is somewhat flexible (such as in a wide canal or comminuted fracture with a gap).

More compelling is the clinical evidence from a prospective randomized controlled trial published in 2024 by Motififard et al. [21], which directly compared exchange nailing versus augmentative plating (with autologous bone grafting) in aseptic femoral shaft nonunions. This multicenter RCT provides high-quality data. The key results at 12 months post-revision were as follows:

- Time to union was significantly shorter in the augmentative plating group (average 5.4 ± 1.3 months) compared to the exchange nailing group (7.4 ± 2.0 months). This was a highly significant difference ($p < 0.001$). Essentially, patients healed about two months faster with the plate strategy.

- Union rate at 12 months: 100% of patients in the plating + graft group achieved union, versus 89.7% in the exchange nailing group. So, while exchange nailing still had a respectable 89.7% union rate, plating achieved virtually 100% union in this trial.

- Clinical outcomes: The plating group had better outcomes on multiple fronts. Operative time was slightly shorter (99 minutes vs. 106 minutes on average), and blood loss was less (about 515 mL vs. 548 mL) in plating compared to nailing, with both differences being statistically significant. Pain relief was greater in the plating group; VAS pain scores dropped from 6 pre-op to 2.6 post-op, whereas in the nailing group, pain went from 5.7 to 3.7. Knee range of motion improved more in the plating group as well. Finally, complication rates were notably different: only approximately 3.6% in plating compared to 17.2% in nailing.

The authors of that RCT concluded that augmentative plating with autologous bone graft is superior to exchange nailing for aseptic femoral shaft nonunions, leading to faster healing, higher union rates, better functional outcomes, and fewer complications [21]. They went so far as to recommend augmentative plating with graft as the preferred treatment option for these cases.

This Level 1 evidence, combined with supportive biomechanical data and prior retrospective studies, is shifting the paradigm in femoral nonunions. Augmentative plating is increasingly seen as the go-to solution, particularly for femur nonunions that might be less likely to respond to a second nail (for example, when the original nail was already large or when the nonunion is at the mid-isthmus, where a nail might still allow rotation). A 2024 meta-analysis of long-bone lower-extremity nonunions after IM nailing [22] found that augmentative plating had higher odds of union (OR ≈ 8.6), shorter union times, less blood loss, and fewer complications than exchange nailing. Subgroup analysis showed shorter union times for augmentative plating in both isthmal and non-isthmal nonunions.

When might exchange nailing still be favored? There are instances where exchange nailing could be the logical choice in the femur:

- If the patient's femoral canal was initially reamed to a small size and a substantially larger nail can now be used, exchange nailing might significantly improve stability.

- If the nonunion has minimal callus and you want the reaming effect to boost biology (though one could ream even with plating by using an RIA graft).

- If there is an infection concern, one might perform an exchange with an antibiotic-coated nail (but that's an infected scenario).

- Patient factors – some might have a strong preference to avoid a plate.

- Surgeon familiarity – not all trauma surgeons are equally comfortable with submuscular plating of the femur.

Other considerations in femoral nonunion surgery:

- Distal femur nonunions: If the nonunion is near the distal metaphysis, a plate might be clearly superior because nails in the distal femur have limited distal fixation, whereas a locking plate can capture distal fragments more effectively.

- Complex femur nonunions: If multiple surgeries have been performed or the bone is very osteoporotic, a plate combined with a nail is sometimes used for additional support.

- Bone grafting: As with the tibia, one nearly always bone grafts atrophic femoral nonunions. In the RCT, the plating group received autograft by protocol, whereas the nailing group presumably did not receive any graft (which might partially explain the higher union rate in the plating group) [21]. This raises an interesting point: Should we also bone graft when performing an exchange nail in the femur? A separate study by Davulcu et al. [23] examined femoral exchange nailing with versus without added bone graft and found no significant difference in union rate or healing time [23]. They concluded that using larger nails is key, and grafting did not significantly change outcomes in their series.

- Compression versus bridge plating: In augmentative plating of the femur, typically one uses a bridge plating technique (spanning the nonunion with a long plate and placing screws only far from the fracture, especially if there is any gap, to avoid disturbing the blood supply). However, since the nail is already *in situ* providing some alignment, some surgeons will perform a so-called "plate-nailing" technique, where they actually compress the nonunion with the plate (if the fracture ends are in contact) to produce axial compression while the nail maintains alignment. Modern locking plates can also be used in compression mode if needed. In hypertrophic nonunions, performing compression with the plate (once fibrous tissue is cleared) can promote direct healing.

- Antibiotic-coated nails: For aseptic nonunions, these are not needed, but it is worth noting that there are intramedullary nails with antibiotic coating (e.g., gentamicin-coated nails) that are mainly used for infected cases, though sometimes prophylactically in high-risk scenarios [10].

Outcomes in femoral nonunion surgery: As illustrated by the RCT, excellent outcomes can be achieved. Augmentative plating has shown nearly 100% union with good functional restoration [21]. Exchange nailing, while slightly less successful in direct comparison, still heals the majority of cases (≈ 85%–90% union). When initial revision fails, subsequent attempts usually succeed. It is rare for a femoral shaft nonunion to persist after multiple properly performed interventions unless infection or massive bone loss is an issue.

Summary for femur: The augmentative plating with nail *in situ* and bone graft approach is emerging as the preferred strategy for aseptic femoral shaft nonunions, given strong evidence of faster and more reliable healing [21]. Exchange nailing remains a viable and historically proven option, especially in cases where plating is less ideal, but evidence now tilts toward plating for most scenarios. Both methods aim to create a stable construct and are often combined with biological enhancement (reaming autograft or iliac crest graft). The specific surgical plan should be individualized. As a final note, patient positioning and approach for femur plating versus nailing differ – exchange nailing is done either supine or lateral on a traction table, usually, while plating often requires a lateral decubitus or supine position with a bump and a fairly large exposure (though sometimes MIPO). With the improved outcomes shown, many orthopedic trauma specialists now recommend augmentative plating (with autograft) as the first-line treatment for a femoral shaft nonunion post-IM nailing, reserving exchange nailing for select cases.

6. Role of bone grafting in nonunion treatment

Bone grafting is a cornerstone of surgical management for atrophic and oligotrophic nonunions, and even in hypertrophic cases, it is often used to speed healing. The fundamental principle is to supply the nonunion site with the biological components that may be lacking: osteogenic cells, osteoinductive factors, and an osteoconductive scaffold. Different types of bone grafts and bone-graft substitutes provide these to varying degrees. Here, we review the main options: autograft (including iliac crest and RIA graft), allograft, and synthetic bone graft extenders or substitutes. We will also touch on specialized grafting techniques, such as vascularized grafts.

Autogenous bone graft (autograft): This remains the gold standard for promoting bone union [24]. Autograft is typically harvested from the patient's own bone, most commonly the iliac crest. It contains living osteogenic cells (osteoblasts and progenitors), osteoinductive growth factors (like BMPs stored in the bone matrix), and provides an osteoconductive scaffold (the bone mineral itself). When placed into a nonunion site, autograft can directly participate in new bone formation and stimulate the host bone to heal. There are two main forms: Cancellous autograft (the spongy medullary bone, which has a high cell and factor content and revascularizes quickly) and cortical autograft (structural pieces of cortical bone, which provide mechanical support but revascularize more slowly). For most nonunions without large segmental defects, cancellous autograft is used because it incorporates and induces healing more rapidly.

The iliac crest (pelvis) is the most common donor site because it has a substantial volume of cancellous bone that is easily accessible. Typically, a surgeon can harvest 30–60 cc of graft from the anterior iliac crest (or more from the posterior crest if needed). Iliac crest bone graft (ICBG) has a very high success record; one reference calls it the "benchmark for the treatment of nonunion regardless of age" [10]. Even in elderly patients, the iliac crest graft still possesses the necessary biology to aid union. Although older patients have fewer stem cells, they still benefit from the graft's osteoconductive and osteoinductive properties.

The downside of autograft is donor site morbidity. Harvesting from the iliac crest can cause significant pain, risk of bleeding, risk of infection, and, rarely, complications like hernia or fracture at the pelvis. Patients often report pain at the crest that can last weeks or months; chronic donor site pain is reported in a minority of patients. Because of these issues, surgeons have sought alternative sources and methods to minimize donor site morbidity.

One such alternative is the RIA system (see **Figures 1–5**), which allows harvesting bone graft from the intramedullary canals (usually the femur, sometimes the tibia) by reaming under suction. The RIA sucks out a paste-like mixture of reamings (which contain bone marrow, small bone fragments, and blood) into a filter trap. This material can yield a large volume of graft (up to 100 cc) rich in marrow elements. RIA graft is essentially intramedullary autograft; it contains marrow MSCs and growth factors, but in a more liquid/cancellous form. Studies have shown RIA graft to have similar union promotion as iliac crest graft for long bone nonunions [25]. The advantage is that there is no separate incision in the pelvis; however, using RIA means you have to access a long bone's canal (which is easy if you are already performing an exchange nailing, for instance). RIA is especially useful in cases with large defects or when you need a lot of graft (such as in the Masquelet

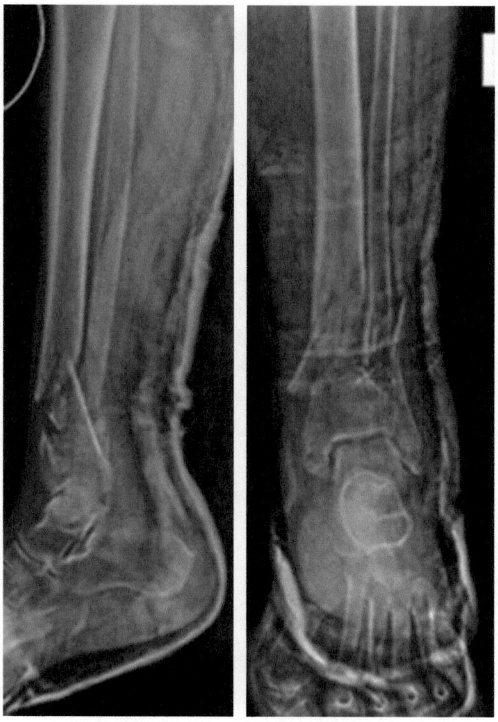

Figure 1.
A 71-year-old female involved in a motor vehicle accident, sustaining multiple traumas including multiple bilateral rib fractures, an open right tibial shaft fracture (Gustilo–Anderson type III), a closed left distal third tibial shaft fracture,, and a closed right mid-shaft femoral fracture.

technique second stage, where you might need 50–100 cc). It also avoids donor site morbidity associated with iliac crest harvest. There are some risks with RIA too; reaming can cause cortical perforation or major bleeding (the RIA flushes fluid, risking fat embolism or hemorrhage if not careful). But overall, it is a well-established technique now.

Another form of autograft is autologous bone marrow aspirate (BMA) or concentrate (BMAC). It involves injecting marrow (with or without concentration) into a nonunion site. While not a "graft" in the structural sense, it is a cellular graft. It has shown good results in some cases and can be used alone or to augment other grafts.

For large structural deficits (>2–3 cm of bone loss), vascularized autografts can be employed. A common example is the free vascularized fibula graft, where a segment of fibula (with its artery and vein) is transplanted to the defect and reconnected via microsurgery to blood vessels near the defect. This provides a living cortical graft with its own blood supply, which can heal into the host bone over time and hypertrophy. Vascularized grafts are complex and usually reserved for scenarios such as atrophic nonunions with massive bone loss or cases where the blood supply of the bed is poor (e.g., after radiation or in a very large defect following tumor resection or infection debridement). In the context of this chapter, for a run-of-the-mill post-traumatic nonunion with a small gap, a vascularized graft is seldom needed; it is more commonly used for limb salvage in extreme cases

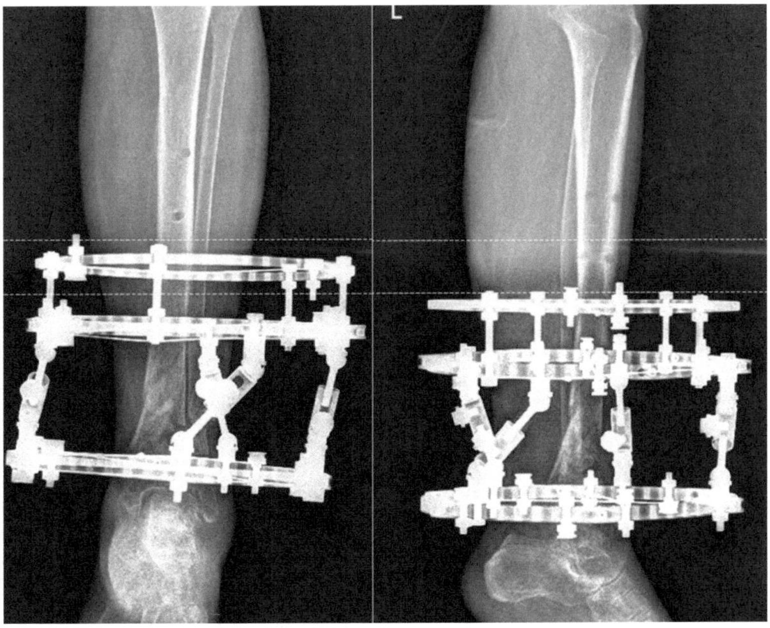

Figure 2.
Sixteen weeks postoperatively, radiographs of the left distal third tibial shaft fracture treated with a circular external fixator (with the foot frame removed at eight weeks postoperatively) demonstrated an absence of visible callus formation and no progression.

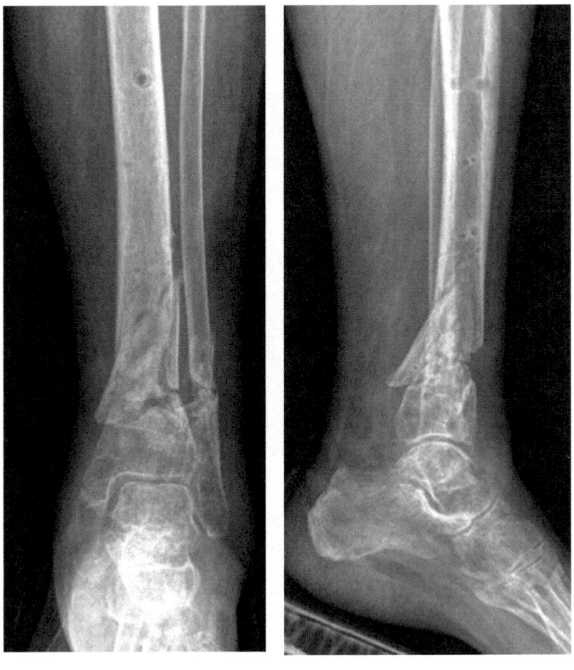

Figure 3.
Five months postoperatively, radiographs demonstrated atrophic nonunion of the distal third of the tibial shaft.

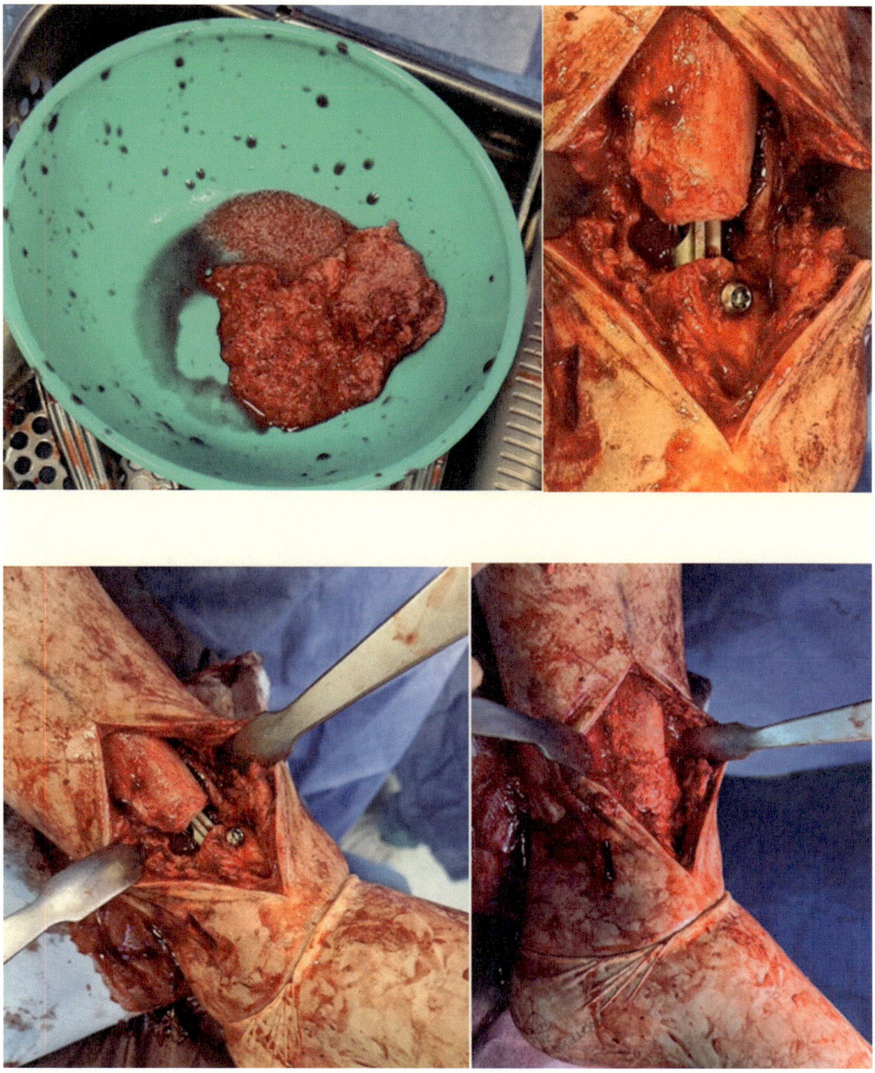

Figure 4.
Intraoperative images showing autologous bone graft harvested using the reamer–irrigator–aspirator (RIA) system, performed retrogradely through the ipsilateral femur, followed by placement of the RIA bone graft into the defect site.

(such as a 10 cm femoral defect). When blood supply is severely compromised, a vascularized graft can succeed where a non-vascularized graft would fail. Vascularized grafts (e.g., fibula) have shown good success but require specialized surgical expertise. Orthopedic references point out that vascularized bone grafts can achieve union in situations of poor blood supply and are the graft of choice in such cases [26]. However, they carry donor site morbidity as well (losing a fibula can slightly affect ankle stability, though usually not significantly if one fibula remains).

Allograft: Allograft refers to bone graft obtained from a donor (cadaver bone, typically processed and stored in a bone bank). It comes in many forms: cortical

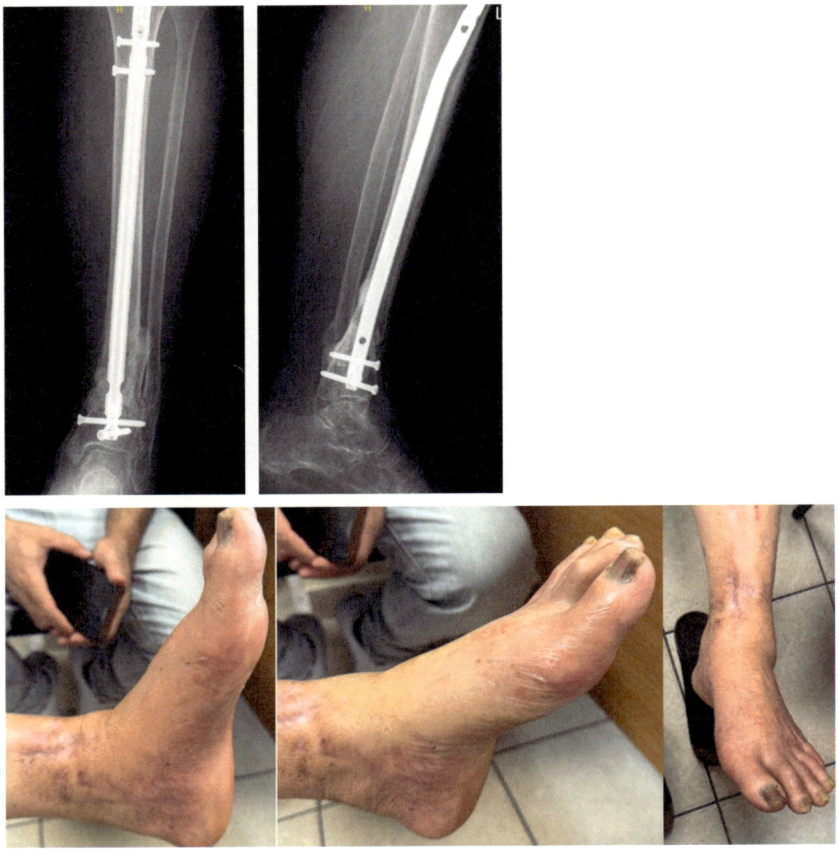

Figure 5.
Nine months postoperatively, the tibial nonunion had achieved complete radiographic union with a good functional outcome; the patient was able to bear full weight without pain.

shafts, corticocancellous chips, morselized cancellous bone, or demineralized bone matrix (DBM; more on that below). Allograft provides a scaffold (osteoconductive), and if not heavily processed, it retains some collagen and proteins that may be mildly osteoinductive. However, it contains no living cells (unless it is a fresh transplant, which is rarely used due to immune reaction). The main advantages of allograft are its availability in large quantities and the avoidance of donor site surgery for the patient. Large structural allografts (like a femoral segment) can be used to bridge massive defects in limb reconstruction. Morselized allograft (freeze-dried chips) is often used as a filler or extender with autograft, for example, mixing autograft 1:1 with cancellous allograft to increase volume.

The downsides include slower incorporation (allograft bone must be slowly remodeled by the host, which can take a long time for large pieces) and the potential for immune response or graft resorption. Disease transmission is extremely low but theoretically possible (modern processing and screening make it very safe, albeit not zero risk). Allograft is often used when autograft is insufficient; for example, in a 5 cm defect after debridement of an infected tibia, one might perform the Masquelet technique and then fill the induced membrane with a mixture of autograft and allograft to achieve sufficient volume. Another scenario: if a patient cannot tolerate autograft harvest (for instance, due to severe osteoporosis or because they have already had their crest harvested previously), one might use allograft chips combined with orthobiologics.

Demineralized bone matrix (DBM): This is a form of allograft that is processed through acid extraction of minerals from cadaver bone, leaving behind the organic collagen matrix and growth factors (notably BMPs) embedded within it. DBM is available as putties or strips. It is primarily osteoinductive (due to BMP content) and osteoconductive (collagen scaffold), but not osteogenic (as it contains no cells). DBM has mild bone-healing capabilities on its own but is usually used as a graft extender (mixed with autograft to spread the autograft further) or as an adjunct to provide some BMP stimulus. Some studies show that DBM alone in a nonunion has limited success, but when combined with autograft, it may enhance the result [25].

Synthetic bone substitutes: These include materials like calcium phosphate ceramics (e.g., hydroxyapatite [HA], tricalcium phosphate), calcium sulfate (plaster of Paris-type materials), bioactive glass, and newer composite scaffolds. Synthetics are osteoconductive scaffolds; they provide a framework for bone growth but usually lack cells or strong inductive factors (unless combined with something like BMP). They come in forms like granules, blocks, or injectable cements. For example, an osteoconductive calcium phosphate cement can be used to fill a bone defect; it hardens, provides immediate structural support, and over time is resorbed and replaced by bone. In nonunion surgery, synthetics can be used to fill residual gaps or augment autograft. One common strategy is to mix synthetic granules with BMA; the synthetic acts as a scaffold, and the marrow brings cells and signals.

Calcium sulfate (e.g., "bone plaster") is sometimes used to fill small defects; it dissolves relatively quickly (within weeks to months) and is fully replaced by bone if everything goes well, but it does not provide long-lasting support. It is more often used as a carrier for antibiotics in infected sites (e.g., Stimulan beads with antibiotics).

Calcium phosphates and HA are more slowly resorbed, providing a scaffold for a longer duration. Some products are even preloaded with collagen or other growth factors. The lack of osteoinductive and osteogenic properties, as well as the high cost of synthetic grafts, has been noted as a concern [10]. They do not contain living cells and typically do not have significant amounts of BMP unless specifically engineered to include it. Therefore, they are usually used as adjuncts rather than as the primary grafts for addressing challenging nonunions.

Graft placement techniques: How the graft is placed also matters. Traditionally, for a stiff atrophic nonunion, surgeons perform an "open decortication and grafting," the nonunion site is fully exposed, all fibrous tissue and sclerosis are removed, and multiple holes are drilled or the cortical bone is scored to induce bleeding (paprika sign) [27]. The area is then packed circumferentially with autograft (sometimes mixed with allograft or DBM) and stabilized with a plate or nail. This creates a local environment rich in osteogenic material.

Special mention – Bone grafting in the presence of infection: In infected nonunions, bone grafting is usually deferred until the infection is controlled (stage 2 of Masquelet or after a period of antibiotic nails, etc.). There are also specialized graft-like techniques, such as the Masquelet-induced membrane technique, where an antibiotic cement spacer is placed in a defect for six to eight weeks to induce a vascularized membrane. The spacer is then removed, and the space is filled with autograft (often combined with allograft/DBM to bulk it) inside that membrane

[26]. This technique has shown good success in treating segmental bone loss of up to 25 cm in some series.

To sum up, the role of bone grafting in nonunions is to re-establish the biology needed for bone healing. Autologous bone (iliac crest or RIA reamings) is the most potent option and is indicated in most atrophic nonunions or any case with bone loss or poor healing potential. It accelerates union and improves union rates significantly [10]. Allografts and synthetic grafts are important adjuncts, particularly when volume is needed or to avoid additional morbidity, but they are usually combined with autograft or orthobiologics for the best results. Ultimately, successful bone grafting requires a well-prepared bed (debridement of scar and sclerotic bone to ensure vascular contact) and stable fixation so that the graft is not extruded and the new vessels can penetrate. When appropriately applied, bone grafts (especially autograft) dramatically improve healing in difficult nonunions, making the difference between persistent failure and successful union in many cases [24].

7. Infection and complex nonunions

Nonunions complicated by infection (septic nonunions) or those with large bone defects and other complexities represent the most challenging subset of cases. They require a tailored approach that addresses both the underlying infection and the lack of bone healing, often necessitating multiple stages of treatment and advanced reconstruction techniques. Infected and complex nonunions typically arise from high-energy open fractures, cases with previous hardware infections, or multiple failed surgeries where biology is severely compromised. Here, we outline strategies for managing these difficult situations.

7.1 Infected nonunions

An infected nonunion means there is persistent osteomyelitis at the fracture site. The dual problem is as given below:

(1) Infection control, eradicating bacteria and infected tissue;

(2) Fracture stabilization and bone healing, achieving union once the site is clean.

These often conflict because infection control might require the removal of hardware and debridement (which destabilizes the bone), and conversely, attempting to stabilize with hardware can introduce surfaces for bacteria to cling to. Thus, careful planning is needed, often in stages.

General principles: As one review aptly stated, infected nonunions present "two interrelated orthopedic problems: deep bone infection and a failure of fracture healing" [28]. The treatment plan must explicitly address both. This usually involves adequate debridement of all infected and nonviable tissues (sequestra, infected bone, scar); culture of tissues to guide antibiotic therapy; stability of the bone (often achieved with external fixation initially, since internal hardware in an infected field is risky until infection is controlled); reconstruction of bone loss (via bone graft, bone transport, or other techniques) once infection is quiescent; and systemic and local antibiotics for a sufficient duration.

Classically, infected nonunions have been treated in stages:

Stage 1: Eradicate infection. Remove any existing hardware (since it harbors biofilm), perform aggressive surgical debridement of the nonunion site (remove all necrotic bone until bleeding healthy bone – the Paprika sign is achieved), collect multiple deep cultures [27], and initiate targeted antibiotic therapy. After debridement, one must maintain stability of the limb; often, an external fixator (e.g., an Ilizarov ring or a unilateral frame) is applied to stabilize the bone after debridement. In some cases, an antibiotic-impregnated cement spacer or an antibiotic cement nail (for intramedullary infection) is placed to deliver a high local antibiotic concentration and maintain some structural support.

Stage 2: Once the infection is under control (typically after a course of 6–12 weeks of antibiotics and confirmation that cultures have become negative and systemic signs have subsided), proceed to definitive reconstruction. This could involve conversion to internal fixation with bone grafting if the infection is eradicated, or bone transport (distraction osteogenesis) using an external fixator to fill any defects, or the Masquelet technique if a large segment has been removed [26].

However, with modern techniques, some cases can be managed in a single stage; for instance, if the infection is low-grade and bone loss is minimal, one might ream out the infection, re-insert a new nail with an antibiotic coating, and concurrently graft. The success of this approach can be good in select cases, but careful patient selection is essential.

Specific strategies:

Antibiotic-coated nails: Intramedullary nails with antibiotic coatings (gentamicin-coated) are now available [29]. These allow one-stage reaming, nail insertion, local antibiotic release, and stability, which can lead to eventual union while treating infection. They are primarily used in femoral or tibial infections. Studies show good infection control and union with these, often obviating the need for a stage with an external fixator.

Ilizarov external fixation (bone transport): For infected nonunions with bone loss, the Ilizarov method is a time-tested solution. After debridement, a circular external fixator is applied. One technique is bone transport, where an osteotomy is created at a healthy bone site (e.g., proximal tibia), and that segment is slowly moved (distracted) across the defect toward the distal segment, generating new bone in the wake [30]. This simultaneously addresses bone loss and avoids large grafts. It is particularly useful if more than 4–5 cm of bone is missing. It also keeps the site open, so if infection flares, additional debridement is possible. The downside is patient discomfort and the long duration in a frame (several months to a year).

Masquelet-induced membrane technique: This two-stage technique has gained popularity for both aseptic and septic segmental bone defects. Stage 1: Place a PMMA antibiotic cement spacer in the bone defect after thorough debridement [26]. This spacer maintains the space and releases antibiotics. The body forms a vascularized membrane around the spacer in four to eight weeks. Stage 2: Remove the spacer and fill the cavity with bone graft (often an autograft + allograft mixture) inside the induced membrane, and stabilize it (either internally or externally). The membrane provides a friendly environment rich in growth factors (like a pseudo-periosteum) that helps the graft consolidate. This technique is effective for defects often up to 25 cm, though large defects may need repeat grafting.

Acute limb shortening and re-lengthening: In some cases, surgeons excise the infected nonunion (removing all compromised bone) and then acutely shorten the limb to bring the bone ends together, addressing the defect by overlap. This approach resolves the gap problem and can eliminate the infection in one step, albeit at the expense of limb length. Subsequently, they gradually lengthen the limb at a different site using an external fixator (similar to performing distraction osteogenesis at the proximal bone). This method addresses both infection and union in one aggressive step; it is particularly considered when soft tissue coverage is problematic or when a very large resection is required (such as acute docking followed by lengthening) [31].

Flap coverage: Many infected nonunions follow open fractures where soft tissue has been damaged. Ensuring good soft tissue coverage is crucial. If a tibial nonunion is open or has scarred skin, bringing in a muscle flap (vascularized muscle or free flap) can help deliver blood supply and antibiotics to the area, aiding in the fight against infection. Flaps (such as a free fibula flap or free muscle flap) can be part of the reconstruction, such as combining a fibula flap for structural support and infection control [32].

Suppression and union-first strategy: There is an approach wherein, if a nonunion is well-fixed and not grossly purulent (just a low-grade infection), one strategy is to suppress the infection with antibiotics (without removing hardware) until union occurs, then remove the hardware and treat osteomyelitis. This is somewhat controversial, but in certain cases (like a minimally symptomatic infection, stable hardware, and good progression of healing), a surgeon might keep the hardware in place, give the patient long-term suppressive antibiotics, allow the fracture to unite, and then remove all hardware and clean out any remaining focus of infection. Some references call this "treat the fracture, then the infection definitively" [33]. This is one strategy out of several. It carries the risk that the infection could worsen but has the benefit of achieving stability and union without destabilizing the construct early.

Outcomes: With comprehensive management, union rates in infected nonunions can still be high (80%–95%), but it often requires multiple surgeries and a prolonged course. The resolution of infection is also high if protocols are followed (most series report > 85% infection eradication, although it sometimes requires more than one debridement). It demands a multidisciplinary approach: collaboration with infectious disease specialists for tailored antibiotic therapy (often six or more weeks of IV antibiotics followed by some oral antibiotics), plastic surgeons for soft tissue coverage, and more. Patience and patient compliance (with external fixator care, avoiding smoking, and maintaining proper nutrition) are critical. Each case is unique; some might be resolved in three months, while others may take 18 months and numerous operations.

7.2 Complex nonunions (large defects, deformities, etc.)

This category often overlaps with infected cases but also includes aseptic cases with significant bone loss or those that have failed multiple surgeries and have poor biology. Examples include a 5 cm segment missing from the femur after a tumor resection (not infected but a complex nonunion scenario), a tibia that has undergone three prior surgeries and is now atrophic, or a nonunion with concurrent issues such as joint contractures or limb length discrepancy.

Large bone defects (aseptic): The strategies mirror those for infection, minus the infection concern. The Masquelet technique is very popular for aseptic defects as well and has shown good success (some studies report ~80%–90% union in large defects) [26]. Bone transport using Ilizarov frames is a classic approach, yielding union in the majority of cases, though the frame time is long (the "rule of thumb": time in frame = 1 month per cm of bone transport plus 2 months, roughly) [30]. Vascularized fibula grafts: For very large defects (>6 cm), some surgeons prefer a free fibula transfer, often combined with a plate for immediate stability. Vascularized fibula can hypertrophy over time and provide a living solution to a large defect, with union at host bone interfaces in ~80% initially, increasing to ~95% after any necessary reoperations [34]. Combinations: For example, plating the bone to bridge a defect with a massive allograft segment and augmenting it with BMP and autograft inside, then hoping it consolidates. Large allografts can incorporate slowly or fracture, but in selected cases (such as a long femoral gap), an allograft segment is one option, often used in tumor reconstructions [35].

Cages or structural scaffolds are employed to bridge large segmental defects, restore anatomical continuity, and provide a stable environment for bone graft incorporation [2]. The treatment of bone loss and nonunion using a cage and autograft is grounded in the principles of mechanical stabilization (via cage or internal fixation) and biological augmentation (using autogenous ICBG), often supplemented by bioregenerative adjuncts (see **Figures 6–9**).

Nonunions with malalignment: Sometimes a nonunion is present alongside a malunion (poor alignment). The revision should address the deformity while also achieving union. Techniques involve performing an osteotomy to realign the bone, followed by fixation with a bone graft. External fixators (e.g., Taylor Spatial Frame) can gradually correct the deformity and compress the nonunion [36], or internal methods can be used with a carefully planned osteotomy. Correcting alignment is crucial because a malaligned nonunion, even if forced to heal, could result in poor function and an increased risk of re-fracture.

Host optimization: Complex nonunions often require addressing patient factors aggressively, for example, metabolic workup (vitamin D, thyroid function, etc.), cessation of NSAIDs, strict no smoking (possibly even using medical therapy like

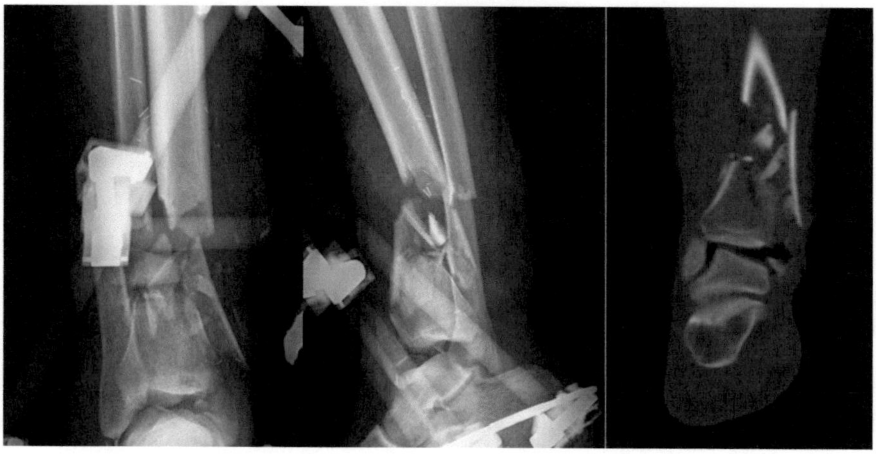

Figure 6.
A 19-year-old male was involved in high-energy motor vehicle accident sustaining multiple traumas including an open comminuted distal tibial fracture (right ankle), classified as Gustilo–Anderson IIIC. Initial management included monoplanar external fixation, wound debridement, and vascular repair of the anterior and posterior tibial arteries in addition to fasciotomy.

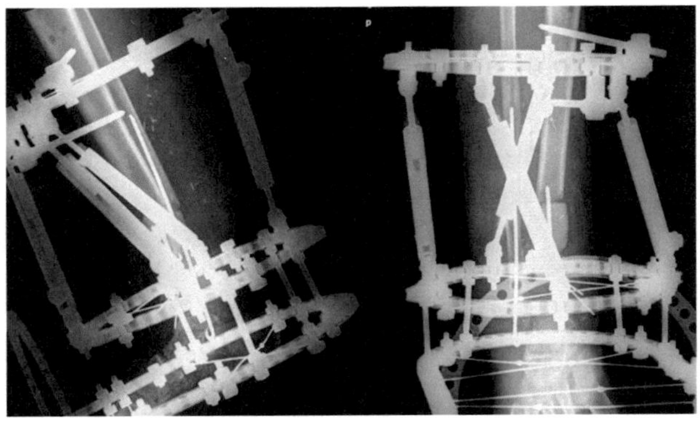

Figure 7.
One month later, the patient underwent circular external fixation (TL-HEX) with resection of 6 cm of distal tibia and placement of vancomycin-loaded cement spacer.

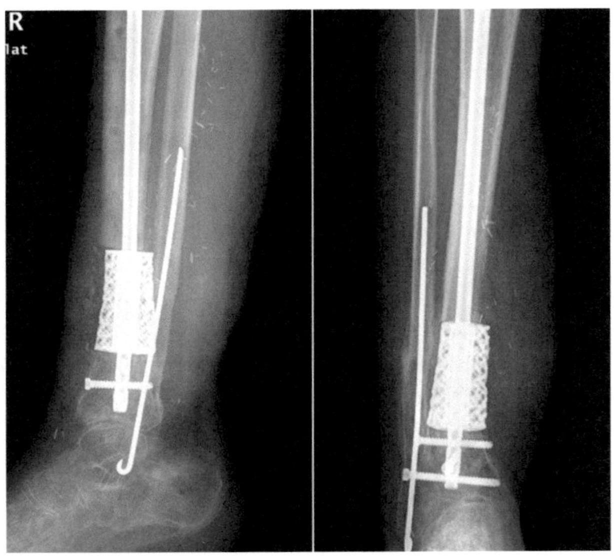

Figure 8.
Five months later, conversion to internal fixation with intramedullary nailing and cage support was performed using an autologous iliac crest bone graft to fill the bone loss.

Chantix to ensure quitting), good nutrition with sufficient protein and possibly supplements (vitamin D, calcium). If the patient has endocrine issues or is on steroids, involvement of an endocrinologist to manage those could improve outcomes [6]. Some centers have "fracture healing clinics" to optimize host physiology.

Adjuvant therapies: In extremely difficult cases, surgeons might throw the kitchen sink; for example, revision with plating, autograft, BMP-2, and then post-op PEMF, and maybe teriparatide for six months. These combined approaches follow the diamond concept to maximize success [6]. It is not always clear which element made the difference, but the goal is to give the bone every chance to heal.

Functional impact and realistic goals: Managing complex and infected nonunions can be a marathon. It is critical to communicate with the patient about the timeline,

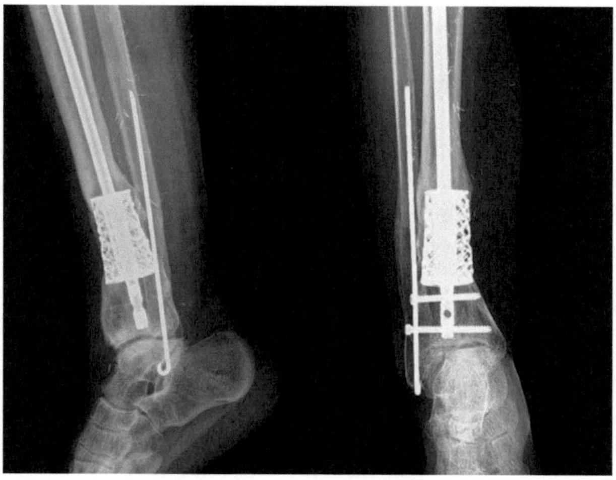

Figure 9.
Four years later, the bone fully healed with good functional outcomes and no signs of infection.

the potential need for multiple procedures, and the expected outcomes. The psychological toll is significant – many such patients have been dealing with a nonunion for a year or more, often with chronic pain and repeated hospitalizations [1]. Psychological support and counseling are important (and often underappreciated) components of care. The surgeon should work with a multidisciplinary team, including physical therapists to maintain joint motion and muscle strength during treatment, plastic surgeons for soft tissue management, and mental health professionals for psychological support [33].

In summary, infected and complex nonunions require an individualized, often staged approach that eradicates infection, provides stability, and reconstructs bone and soft tissues. Successful outcomes are attainable, with reported union rates often exceeding 85% after comprehensive treatment, but achieving these outcomes requires significant time and resources. This underscores the importance of specialized centers (limb reconstruction centers) for these cases, as evidence shows that such multidisciplinary teams improve outcomes with fewer complications [30]. Patience and perseverance from both the surgeon and the patient are key, as is the willingness to adapt the plan if one method fails (having a plan B, C, or D as needed).

8. Summary and recommendations

Fracture nonunion of the tibia or femur is a complex but treatable condition. Through advances in both surgical techniques and adjuvant therapies, orthopedic surgeons today can achieve union in the vast majority of cases, even those that historically might have resulted in amputation or permanent disability. This chapter has detailed the multifactorial nature of nonunions and the array of tools available to address them. Here, we distill key points and provide practical recommendations:

- Early identification and classification: Distinguish delayed healing from nonunion early. If a tibial or femoral fracture shows no progress by four to six months, begin evaluation for causes of nonunion. Use a pragmatic definition: Any fracture that will not heal without intervention should be considered a nonunion. Classify the nonunion by radiographic appearance (hypertrophic, oligotrophic, atrophic) and by whether infection is present. This guides treatment: Hypertrophic typically means stability is the issue, atrophic means biology is lacking, and infection changes the entire algorithm. Always investigate for occult infection in "aseptic" nonunions (get cultures intra-op), a routine advocated by Mills et al. [5].

- Address all contributing factors (mechanical and biological): Successful nonunion treatment requires correcting mechanical instability and enhancing the biological environment. This "dual requirement" is encapsulated in the Diamond Concept [6]. In practice:

    - Mechanical: Provide adequate stability through internal fixation (plate or nail) or external fixation. In tibial nonunions, both exchange nailing and plate-over-nail yield high union rates; choose based on patient factors and surgeon expertise. Meta-analytic data suggest that augmentative plating can offer higher union odds and shorter healing times in long-bone nonunions overall [22]. For most femoral nonunions, we recommend augmentative compression plating with autologous bone graft as the first-line revision strategy, given its faster union and higher success rates.

    - Biological: Atrophic nonunions need aggressive biological enhancement. Perform thorough decortication of the nonunion site, removing sclerotic bone and interposed fibrous tissue until punctate bleeding bone is seen (paprika sign) [4]. Then, add autologous bone graft (iliac crest or RIA reamings) liberally, as it remains the gold standard osteogenic material [24]. Consider adjuvants like BMP-2 or BMP-7 in refractory cases or when autograft is limited; they have been shown to significantly improve union rates and can substitute for autograft in certain scenarios [2].

- Infection control: If infection is present or suspected, prioritize its management. Our recommendation is a staged approach: Stage 1 – debride thoroughly and eradicate infection using external fixation or an antibiotic-coated nail for provisional stability, and administer targeted antibiotics (guided by cultures) for at least six to eight weeks [37]. Stage 2 – reconstruct after confirming infection clearance (normalized CRP, good soft tissue healing). Reconstruction may involve internal fixation and grafting or bone transport/Masquelet technique for large defects [26]. Alternatively, consider one-stage strategies in select cases using antibiotic-coated implants if tissue conditions allow – but be prepared to convert to a multi-stage approach if any doubt remains. Always obtain multiple deep cultures at the time of nonunion surgery (even if considered aseptic) to detect latent infection [38].

- Use evidence-based fixation strategies: For femoral shaft nonunions after nailing, the latest Level I evidence clearly supports augmentative plating with autograft over exchange nailing [21]. We therefore advise augmentative locked plating (4.5 mm plate) applied over a retained nail with concurrent autograft for femoral nonunions, especially those with any rotational instability or those that have already undergone one failed nailing. The biomechanical superiority and clinical success (100% union in RCT) make it the preferred option. Either approach is acceptable; if one method fails, the other can serve as a backup. Locking plates spanning the nonunion combined with intramedullary stability (either nail *in situ* or fibular graft) provide excellent outcomes and should be part of the armamentarium.

- Adjunctive stimulation: Consider employing bone stimulators as adjuncts, particularly in situations where additional surgery is risky or as a complement post-surgery. We recommend LIPUS (20 minutes daily) for delayed unions or as an adjunct after revision fixation of an atrophic nonunion, given that LIPUS is safe, although unsupported by strong evidence [12]. Likewise, PEMF therapy (eight hours daily) is an effective adjunct or standalone treatment, with healing rates of approximately 75%–85% in long bone nonunions [11]. For example, in a patient who is a poor surgical candidate or refuses surgery, a trial of PEMF is warranted and often successful in achieving union over several months. Even after surgical fixation, there is minimal downside to adding a PEMF device to "hedge" against another nonunion, especially in biologically tenuous cases. Ensure patient compliance with these devices, as their effectiveness depends on regular use.

- Plan for bone loss and complex reconstruction: In cases of significant bone loss or segmental defects (common in high-energy tibial injuries), anticipate the need for advanced techniques:

    - For defects measuring 1–5 cm, the Masquelet-induced membrane technique is a reliable two-stage option. We recommend this method for managing contained defects: Stage one involves an antibiotic spacer, and stage two utilizes an autograft/allograft filler with stable fixation. This approach has demonstrated high union rates, even in infected scenarios [26].

    - If the defect is larger or if limb length is a concern, use Ilizarov external fixation for bone transport. Although lengthy, it can restore both length and continuity without a graft (especially useful if infection precludes large grafting) [30].

    - Consider vascularized bone grafts (e.g., free fibula flap) for very challenging defects or when the regional blood supply is poor. These grafts bring live bone and blood supply and have excellent success in experienced hands for bridging massive gaps [34].

    - Always involve plastic or reconstructive surgeons early if soft tissue coverage is an issue – a well-vascularized soft tissue envelope is paramount for both infection control and bone healing. A muscle flap can be as important as the bone work in some cases [6].

- Psychosocial support: Do not overlook the psychological impact. Nonunion patients often endure chronic pain, loss of function, and social role changes (e.g., inability to work, financial stress). Depression and anxiety are common.

We recommend incorporating mental health evaluation and support as part of nonunion care [1]. This might involve counseling, support groups (some find solace in hearing other patients' journeys), or appropriate medications if needed. As the clinician, maintain a positive yet realistic outlook with the patient. Reassure them that union is achievable (e.g., "With the plan we have, there's over a 90% chance your bone will heal," is encouraging) but also prepare them for the commitment and possible hurdles. Setting expectations about treatment duration and potential setbacks helps patients cope better and adhere to the plan.

- Multidisciplinary approach: Whenever possible, treat nonunions in specialized centers or teams that include orthopedic trauma/reconstructive surgeons, plastic surgeons, infectious disease specialists, physiatrists, and so on. The evidence and our experience suggest that a multidisciplinary, comprehensive approach yields the best outcomes in complex nonunions [33]. This ensures each aspect (bone, soft tissue, infection, rehabilitation, psychological) is optimally managed. Regular team meetings to review progress can be useful for complex cases.

- In conclusion, successful management of tibial and femoral nonunions hinges on identifying and correcting all factors inhibiting healing, from providing rigid fixation and viable bone grafts, to controlling infection and optimizing patient health. The combination of modern fixation methods (particularly augmentative plating for long bone nonunions), advanced bone grafting and orthobiologic adjuncts, and dedicated patient care has made even the most stubborn nonunions curable in most instances. By following evidence-based strategies and tailoring them to each patient's unique situation, orthopedic surgeons can expect high union rates and restored function. Always remember the aphorism: "The only failure in nonunion treatment is failure to address the cause of the nonunion." By thoroughly addressing mechanical stability, biological vitality, and host factors, the cause(s) of nonunion are removed, and successful bone healing will follow.

Conflict of Interest

The authors declare no conflict of interest.

Author details

Khalil Nasrallah*, Fadi Abboud, Einal Bathish and Haim Shtarker
Galilee Medical Center, Nahariya, Israel

*Address all correspondence to: kn171010@gmail.com

References

[1] Brinker MR, Hanus BD, Sen M, O'Connor DP. The devastating effects of tibial nonunion on health-related quality of life. The Journal of Bone and Joint Surgery – American Volume. 2013;**95**(24):2170–6. DOI: 10.2106/JBJS.L.00803

[2] Calori GM, Albisetti W, Agus A, Iori S, Tagliabue L. Risk factors contributing to fracture non-unions. Injury. 2007;**38** (Suppl 2):S11–8. DOI: 10.1016/s0020-1383(07)80004-0

[3] Jin YF, Xu HC, Shen ZH, Pan XK, Xie H. Comparing augmentative plating and exchange nailing for the treatment of nonunion of femoral shaft fracture after intramedullary nailing: A meta-analysis. Orthopaedic Surgery. 2020;**12**(1):50–57. DOI: 10.1111/os.12580

[4] Weber, B. G, and Oldřich Čech. Pseudarthrosis : Pathophysiology, Biomechanics, Therapy, Results. New York: Grune & Stratton; 1976

[5] Mills, L. A., Aitken, S. A., & Simpson, A. H. R. W.. The risk of non-union per fracture: Current myths and revised figures from a population of over 4 million adults. Acta Orthopaedica. 2017;**88**(4):434–439. DOI: 10.1080/17453674.2017.1321351

[6] Giannoudis PV, Einhorn TA, Marsh D. Fracture healing: The diamond concept. Injury. 2007;**38**(Suppl 4):S3–S6

[7] Wang L, Tower RJ, Chandra A, Yao L, Tong W, Xiong Z, Tang K, Zhang Y, Liu XS, Boerckel JD, Guo X, Ahn J, Qin L. Periosteal mesenchymal progenitor dysfunction and extraskeletally-derived fibrosis contribute to atrophic fracture nonunion. Journal of Bone and Mineral Research. 2019;**34**(3):520–532. DOI: 10.1002/jbmr.3626

[8] Scolaro JA, Schenker ML, Yannascoli S, Baldwin K, Mehta S, Ahn J. Cigarette smoking increases complications following fracture: A systematic review. Journal of Bone and Joint Surgery. 2014;**96**(8):674–681. DOI: 10.2106/JBJS.M.00081

[9] Brinker MR, O'Connor DP. Exchange nailing of ununited fractures. The Journal of Bone and Joint Surgery – American Volume. 2007;**89**(1):177–88. DOI: 10.2106/JBJS.F.00742

[10] Papakostidis C, Kanakaris NK, Pretel J, Faour O, Morell DJ, Giannoudis PV. Prevalence and management of femoral and tibial nonunion. Bone & Joint Research. 2015;**5**(12):512–523

[11] Aaron RK, Ciombor DM, Simon BJ. Treatment of nonunions with electric and electromagnetic fields. Clinical Orthopaedics and Related Research. 2004;**419**:21–29

[12] Busse JW, Kaur J, Mollon B, Bhandari M, Tornetta P 3rd, Schünemann HJ, Guyatt GH. Low intensity pulsed ultrasonography for fractures: Systematic review of randomised controlled trials. BMJ. 2009;**338**:b351. DOI: 10.1136/bmj.b351

[13] Aspenberg P, Genant HK, Johansson T, Nino AJ, See K, Krohn K, Mitlak BH. Teriparatide for acceleration of fracture repair in humans: A prospective, randomized, double-blind study of 102 postmenopausal women with distal

radial fractures. Journal of Bone and Mineral Research. 2010;**25**(2): 404–414

[14] Swanson ER, Garrard EC, Bernstein DT, O'Connor DP, Brinker MR. Results of a systematic approach to exchange nailing for the treatment of aseptic femoral nonunions. Journal of Orthopaedic Trauma. 2015;**29**(1):21–7. DOI:10.1097/BOT.0000000000000166

[15] Le Baron M, Vivona JP, Maman P, Volpi R, Flecher X. Can the reamer/irrigator/aspirator system replace anterior iliac crest grafting when treating long bone nonunion? Orthopaedics & Traumatology: Surgery & Research. 2019;**105**(3):529–533. DOI: 10.1016/j.otsr.2018.12.011

[16] Birjandinejad A, Ebrahimzadeh MH, Ahmadzadeh-Chabock H. Augmentation plate fixation for the treatment of femoral and tibial nonunion after intramedullary nailing. Orthopedics. 2009;**32**(6):409. DOI: 10.3928/01477447-20090511-12

[17] Wiss DA, Stetson WB. Unstable fractures of the tibia treated with a reamed intramedullary interlocking nail. Clinical Orthopaedics and Related Research. 1995;**315**:56–63

[18] Baldwin P, Li DJ, Auston DA, Mir HS, Yoon RS, Koval KJ. Autograft, allograft, and bone graft substitutes: Clinical evidence and indications for use in the setting of orthopaedic trauma surgery. Journal of Orthopaedic Trauma. 2019;**33**(4): 203–213. DOI: 10.1097/BOT.0000000000001420

[19] Bleeker NJ, van de Wall BJM, IJpma FFA, Doornberg JN, Kerkhoffs GMMJ, Jaarsma RL, Knobe M, Link BC, Babst R, Beeres FJP. Plate vs. nail for extra-articular distal tibia fractures: How should we personalize surgical treatment? A meta-analysis of 1332 patients. Injury. 2021;**52**(3):345–357. DOI: 10.1016/j.injury.2020.10.026

[20] Walcher MG, Day RE, Gesslein M, Bail HJ, Kuster MS. Augmentative plating versus exchange intramedullary nailing for the treatment of aseptic non-unions of the femoral shaft-A biomechanical study in a SawboneTM model. Journal of Personalized Medicine. 2023;**13**(4):650. DOI: 10.3390/jpm13040650

[21] Motififard M, Mousavi H, Iranpanah N, Akbari Aghdam H, Teimouri M, Aliakbari M, Parhamfar M, Shirazi Nejad S, Shahsavan M, Daemi A, Salehi A, Shahsavan M. Comparative study of exchange nailing and augmentative plating for treating aseptic nonunion of femoral shafts post intramedullary nailing: A single-blind, multicentric randomized clinical trial. Journal of Clinical Medicine. 2024;**13** (22):6928. DOI: 10.3390/jcm13226928

[22] Fu CX, Gao H, Ren J, Wang H, Lu SK, Wang GL, Zhu ZF, Liu YY, Luo W, Zhang Y, Zhang YF. Effectiveness and safety of augmentative plating technique in managing nonunion following intramedullary nailing of long bones in the lower extremity: A systematic review and meta-analysis. Chinese Journal of Traumatology. 2025;**28**(3):164–174. DOI: 10.1016/j.cjtee.2024.04.004

[23] Davulcu CD, Saruhan S, Bilgin E, Zengin EC. Effect of bone grafting on bone union in exchange nailing for the treatment of femoral shaft nonunions. Northern Clinics of Istanbul. 2024;**11**(4): 322–327. DOI: 10.14744/nci.2023.43410

[24] Giannoudis PV, Dinopoulos H, Tsiridis E. Bone substitutes: An update. Injury. 2005;**36**(Suppl 3):S20–S27

[25] Giannoudis PV, Tzioupis C, Green J. Surgical techniques: how I do it? The Reamer/Irrigator/Aspirator (RIA) system. Injury. 2009;**40**(11):1231–6. DOI: 10.1016/j.injury.2009.07.070

[26] Masquelet AC, Giannoudis PV. The induced membrane technique for treatment of bone defects: What have I learned? Trauma Case Reports. 2021;**36**: 100556. DOI: 10.1016/j.tcr.2021.100556

[27] Müller ME, Allgöwer M, Willenegger H. Manual of Internal Fixation: Techniques Recommended by the AO Group. Berlin: Springer-Verlag; 1979

[28] Motsitsi NS. Management of infected nonunion of long bones: The last decade (1996–2006). Injury. 2008;**39**(2):155–160

[29] Fuchs T, Stange R, Schmidmaier G, Raschke MJ. The use of gentamicin-coated nails in the tibia: Preliminary results of a prospective study. Archives of Orthopaedic and Trauma Surgery. 2011;**131**(10):1419–1425

[30] Catagni MA, Azzam W, Guerreschi F, Lovisetti L, Poli P, Khan MS, Di Giacomo LM. Trifocal versus bifocal bone transport in treatment of long segmental tibial bone defects. The Bone & Joint Journal. 2019;**101-B** (2):162–169. DOI: 10.1302/0301-620X.101B2.BJJ-2018-0340.R2

[31] Cattaneo R, Catagni M, Johnson EE. The treatment of infected nonunions and segmental defects of the tibia by the methods of Ilizarov. Clinical Orthopaedics and Related Research. 1992;**280**:143–52

[32] Godina M. Early microsurgical reconstruction of complex trauma of the extremities. Plastic and Reconstructive Surgery. 1986;**78**(3):285–292

[33] Calori GM, Phillips M, Jeetle S, Tagliabue L, Giannoudis PV. Classification of non-union: Need for a new scoring system? Injury. 2007;**39** (Suppl 2):S59–S63

[34] Hanba C, Lin TC, Wei FC. The fibula osteoseptocutaneous flap: evolution in concepts, techniques, and technologies during mandibular reconstruction - A review. International Journal of Surgery. 2024;**110**(11): 7196–7201. DOI: 10.1097/JS9.0000000000001972

[35] Bus MP, Dijkstra PD, van de Sande MA, Taminiau AH, Schreuder HW, Jutte PC, van der Geest IC, Schaap GR, Bramer JA. Intercalary allograft reconstructions following resection of primary bone tumors: A nationwide multicenter study. Journal of Bone and Joint Surgery. 2014;**96**(4):e26. DOI: 10.2106/JBJS.M.00655

[36] Paley, D. Principles of deformity correction. Berlin: Springer; 2002

[37] Metsemakers WJ, et al. Infection after fracture fixation: Current surgical and microbiological concepts. Injury 2019;**50**:1642–1649

[38] Wagner RK, Emmelot MP, van Trikt C, Visser CE, Peters EJG, Janssen SJ, Kloen P. Characteristics and Outcomes of Occult Infections in Presumed Aseptic Nonunions: A Retrospective Cohort Study. Journal of Orthopaedic Trauma. 2024;**38**(8):452–458. DOI: 10.1097/BOT.0000000000002822

Chapter 7

Current Strategies in the Management of Complicated Fractures

Murat Yüncü

Abstract

The treatment paradigm for complex fractures has transformed into a multidisciplinary framework that integrates mechanical stability, soft-tissue preservation, and patient-specific optimization. High-energy injuries frequently complicate management due to extensive comminution, significant soft-tissue compromise, and an elevated risk of infection. Contemporary strategies emphasize biological osteosynthesis and minimally invasive fixation techniques, aiming to preserve vascularity, minimize iatrogenic trauma, and enhance the intrinsic healing environment. The incorporation of digital technologies – including preoperative three-dimensional (3D) planning, patient-specific implants, and computer-assisted reduction – has further refined surgical precision, improving reduction quality and reducing operative morbidity. Infection prevention remains a central priority in the management of these injuries. Early antibiotic prophylaxis, timely and thorough debridement, and coordinated orthoplastic collaboration substantially reduce postoperative complications. Standardized diagnostic criteria and structured multidisciplinary team (MDT) decision-making are essential components in the treatment of fracture-related infection. Moreover, orthobiologic interventions such as mesenchymal stem cells, platelet-rich plasma, and bone morphogenetic proteins have expanded therapeutic options, particularly in challenging cases of delayed union and nonunion, by enhancing the biological potential for regeneration. In geriatric patients, individualized care pathways incorporating metabolic optimization, principles of fragility fracture management, and orthogeriatric co-management have been shown to reduce complications and facilitate early mobilization. Overall, the modern approach to complex fractures is defined by the integration of biology, biomechanics, and clinical reasoning. This chapter provides a comprehensive and up-to-date overview of these evolving concepts, highlighting the ongoing shift toward personalized, biologically attuned, and multidisciplinary trauma care.

Keywords: complex fractures, biological osteosynthesis, multidisciplinary trauma care, fracture-related infection, orthobiologics, 3D-assisted surgery

1. Introduction

1.1 General framework

The management of complex fractures is one of the most intricate areas of orthopedic trauma. Comminuted fractures resulting from high-energy trauma, with their associated risks of bone loss, soft tissue disruption, and infection, continue to challenge the boundaries of both surgical technique and biological understanding [1]. Despite advancements in fixation techniques, implant design, and imaging methods, complications such as delayed union, nonunion, and infection remain significant obstacles to achieving successful outcomes.

1.2 Clinical significance of infection and treatment paradigm

Rupp et al. [2] reported that infection following a fracture remains a leading cause of treatment failure and prolonged morbidity in long bone fractures. This situation reiterates the need for integrated, multidisciplinary approaches that target both mechanical and biological healing.

1.3 Multidisciplinary framework and the rising biological focus in fracture-related infection management

The management of fracture-related infection (FRI) requires not only meticulous surgical debridement and implant handling but also a coordinated multidisciplinary framework that integrates orthopedic trauma, plastic surgery, and infectious disease expertise. Metsemakers et al. [1] emphasized that FRI should be regarded as an independent clinical entity with standardized diagnostic criteria, forming the basis for contemporary evidence-based treatment protocols worldwide.

In recent years, fracture treatment strategies have undergone a fundamental paradigm shift – from purely mechanical reconstruction toward biologically conscious fixation. Earlier generations of trauma surgeons often prioritized anatomical reduction through extensive surgical exposures, frequently compromising periosteal perfusion and soft-tissue integrity. In contrast, modern principles such as biological osteosynthesis, minimally invasive percutaneous plate osteosynthesis (MIPO), and the safe definitive surgery (SDS) concept prioritize the preservation of the biological environment alongside stable fixation.

Kalbas et al. [3] reported that physiologically guided surgical timing within safe and definitive limits reduces systemic stress, shortens hospitalization, and significantly decreases postoperative complication rates in polytrauma patients. This evolving philosophy underscores that a fracture environment is not merely a structural defect within bone, but rather a dynamic biological ecosystem – an interplay of cellular, vascular, and systemic factors that collectively determine the capacity for healing.

1.4 Fracture biology: Osteogenesis, angiogenesis, and mechanotransduction

Studies indicate that current biological findings regarding the processes of osteogenesis and angiogenesis more clearly demonstrate the effects of mechanical stimuli, oxygen tension, and immune signaling on callus formation. The review by

Hoang et al. [4] regarding stem cell-mediated bone repair highlighted the role of mesenchymal stem cells (MSCs) as multipotent regulatory cells, demonstrating that these cells respond to local microenvironmental cues and link mechanical stability to molecular repair mechanisms.

1.5 Digital planning and personalized implant engineering

The contemporary management of complex fractures is shaped by a multidimensional framework arising from the convergence of multiple disciplines, advanced technologies, and evolving insights in biological sciences. Liang et al. [5] demonstrated that the integration of three-dimensional (3D) printing and computer-assisted design enables surgeons to fabricate patient-specific plates that conform precisely to individual anatomy, thereby minimizing intraoperative adjustments and preserving soft-tissue integrity. This advancement represents a paradigm shift from the traditional "one-size-fits-all" fixation philosophy toward truly personalized trauma care.

Ling et al. [6] quantitatively validated these benefits, showing that 3D-assisted fracture surgery reduces operative time and intraoperative blood loss by approximately 30%, while improving radiological alignment by 20%–25%. Furthermore, preoperative digital modeling allows surgeons to anticipate potential implant conflicts, minimize soft-tissue dissection, and enhance the accuracy of screw placement. Collectively, these findings illustrate how digital planning and additive manufacturing technologies are progressively transforming orthopedics into a precision engineering discipline.

Castillón et al. [7] specifically emphasized the biomechanical importance of implant overlap in the treatment of fractures in previously implant-fixed femurs. While direct experimental evidence is lacking, the general consensus in the literature suggests that maintaining continuity between old and new implants can reduce stress concentration, potentially reducing the risk of re-fracture.

These conceptual considerations clearly demonstrate the growing understanding of fracture biomechanics and the need to design surgical strategies consistent with biological principles.

1.6 Mechano-biological balance and fixation philosophy

The concept of mechanical–biological balance underlies these strategies. Fracture healing is achieved not only through rigid fixation but also by creating an optimal stress environment that maintains vascular integrity while stimulating callus formation. Bowers et al. [8] stated that excessive mechanical stiffness delays the healing process by suppressing osteogenic signaling; conversely, controlled micromobility promotes bone remodeling through mechanotransduction [8, 9]. Implant designs that provide variable stiffness and allow for load sharing, such as locking plate systems that function as internal fixators, are a concrete reflection of the evolving concept of aligning mechanical design with physiological requirements.

1.7 Smart fixation and sensor-based monitoring

The concept of "smart fixation" places the surgeon in the role of both engineer and biologist. Therefore, mechanical conditions must be optimized according to biological potential. In recent years, integrated fixation devices with sensors that simultaneously monitor mechanical load and micromobility have become available [10]. Artificial Wi–Fi-based applications within these "smart implants" allow for early detection of implant loosening or rupture delay by analyzing feedback loops, ushering in a new era of data-driven orthopedic initiation.

1.8 Infection prophylaxis and the integrated orthoplastic approach

Infection prevention and control remain fundamental components in the management of complex fractures. Despite the availability of advanced antibiotics and biomaterials, infection rates in high-grade open fractures remain clinically significant. Whiting et al. [11] emphasized the critical importance of antibiotic timing, reporting that the administration of intravenous antibiotics within the first hour after injury markedly reduces bacterial colonization and, consequently, the risk of infection.

Beyond systemic therapy, contemporary strategies highlight the value of local antibiotic delivery. Methods such as vancomycin powder application or antibiotic-impregnated calcium sulfate beads maintain high local antibiotic concentrations while minimizing systemic toxicity [12]. Roberts et al. [13] demonstrated that an orthoplastic collaborative model, in which debridement, skeletal fixation, and soft-tissue reconstruction are planned and executed simultaneously, significantly decreases reinfection rates and accelerates wound healing.

Collectively, these findings reflect a paradigm shift in trauma management, from sequential treatment protocols toward integrated and synchronized care models that align surgical precision with biological preservation.

1.9 Multidisciplinary team processes and decision-making

Furthermore, the multidisciplinary methodology proposed by Metsemakers et al. [1] emphasizes the importance of early multidisciplinary team (MDT) consultation in determining prognosis. Infection control, bone stability, and host immunity are not independent variables; rather, they are interrelated biological processes that must be addressed through a comprehensive and coordinated approach. One of the most defining characteristics of contemporary complex fracture management lies precisely within this multidisciplinary framework.

Hutchinson et al. [14] reported that structured MDT meetings involving trauma surgeons, infectious disease specialists, and plastic surgeons enhance diagnostic accuracy, facilitate surgical planning, and improve limb salvage rates. The MDT approach ensures that decision-making remains dynamic and patient-centered, considering not only fracture morphology but also systemic stability, nutritional status, and psychosocial factors influencing recovery.

Rupp et al. [2] further noted that regular team-based case discussions enable early detection of complications, such as implant failure or delayed union, allowing timely intervention. Consequently, the management of complex fractures has evolved from a single-surgeon-driven model into a collaborative, algorithm-guided process supported by collective expertise.

1.10 Orthobiologic approaches and host optimization

Similarly, a transformative advancement has emerged in the field of orthobiologic agents and regenerative medicine. Impieri et al. [15] investigated the use of biologic adjuvants such as bone morphogenetic proteins (BMPs), platelet-rich plasma (PRP), and MSCs, concluding that these agents can significantly accelerate fracture healing when combined with stable fixation and appropriate mechanical stimulation.

Expanding on this concept, Bin Shahri et al. [16] demonstrated that MSCs secrete pro-osteogenic cytokines, such as vascular endothelial growth factor (VEGF) and transforming growth factor-beta (TGF-β), which enhance angiogenesis and callus mineralization in both upper and lower extremity nonunions. Moreover, the authors emphasized that the efficacy of orthobiologic interventions reaches its maximum when applied in a mechanically stable and infection-free environment, thereby reinforcing the principle of "biology supported by biomechanics."

At the molecular level, Hoang et al. [4] provided further insights, showing that MSCs modulate macrophage polarization and reduce chronic inflammation, thereby elucidating the link between immune regulation and bone regeneration. When combined with host optimization strategies such as glycemic control, vitamin D correction, and smoking cessation, these treatments offer a biologically integrated roadmap toward functional recovery and long-term skeletal restoration.

1.11 Management in geriatric and osteoporotic patients

The growing number of elderly trauma patients has redefined the dynamics of complex fracture management. Fragility fractures, characterized by osteoporotic bone structure and reduced healing capacity, demand both surgical innovation and systemic support.

Welzel et al. [17] reported that, in geriatric patients with periarticular fractures, the use of personalized fixation techniques combining locking-plate technology with pharmacologic bone-strengthening agents, such as teriparatide and vitamin D supplementation, proved beneficial. In their multicenter orthogeriatric study, coordinated co-management between trauma and geriatric teams was shown to reduce postoperative delirium rates and improve mobility scores at discharge [17].

Prioritizing functional restoration over anatomical perfection reflects a pragmatic paradigm shift, one that recognizes quality of life and independence as primary outcomes in the management of elderly and osteoporotic fracture patients.

1.12 Continuity of care and patient-centered outcomes

This patient-centered perspective is gaining increasing importance in modern orthopedic trauma care. Mere survival is no longer considered sufficient; the ultimate goal is reintegration into daily life and the restoration of lasting functional independence.

When viewed collectively, these advancements reveal that fracture management has evolved from a purely mechanical craft into a restorative science that integrates biology, engineering, and multidisciplinary collaboration. Complex fractures are no longer perceived as isolated events but rather as manifestations of systemic imbalance between biological integrity, mechanical stability, and host resilience.

The future of this field lies in the seamless integration of technology, regenerative biology, and team-based care, each reinforcing the other to achieve infection-free union and optimal functional recovery. As emphasized collectively by Metsemakers [1], Bin Shahri [16], Ling [6], and Welzel [17], the key to success in fracture management lies not in the sophistication of implants but in the wisdom with which they are applied – recognizing that every fracture is not merely a mechanical disruption but a biological event that demands systemic harmony.

2. Development

2.1 General framework and goals

Treatment of complex fractures requires a precise balance between surgical precision, respect for biological tissue, and multidisciplinary coordination. Once the acute stabilization phase of the injury is complete, the focus should shift to optimizing both mechanical reconstruction and the biological environment necessary for bone healing. The ultimate goal is to achieve stable fixation without disrupting soft tissue integrity, minimize the risk of infection, and promote early functional recovery. Therefore, the modern trauma surgeon must function not only as a technical practitioner but also as a "physiological systems orchestrator," who orchestrates mechanical correction in harmony with cellular and vascular biology.

2.2 The principle of biological osteosynthesis (respect for tissue)

Central to this process is the concept of biological osteosynthesis, which is based on the principle that fractures heal best when the natural biology of the bone is preserved and supported. Extensive periosteal stripping and disruption of vascular channels, commonly used in open reduction procedures in the past, are now recognized as factors that negatively impact healing. MIPO and bridge plating techniques have largely replaced traditional open surgical approaches for comminuted and metaphyseal fractures [18]. Beeharry et al. [19] demonstrated that minimizing surgical trauma and preserving the fracture hematoma with the MIPO technique accelerates callus formation and reduces infection rates. This principle of "respect for biology" forms the cornerstone of modern fixation, emphasizing that the surgeon's role should focus on providing optimal biological conditions for the natural repair process rather than establishing rigid mechanical superiority.

2.3 Locking plate systems and variable stiffness

Locking plate systems represent one of the most concrete examples of the biological osteosynthesis approach. These systems function as internal fixators, providing angular stability while maintaining periosteal blood flow. By allowing controlled micromobility, they promote callus formation and support secondary bone healing. However, Bowers et al. [8] reported that excessively rigid constructs can suppress mechanical stimulation, resulting in delayed union or nonunion. Therefore, developing variable stiffness implants aims to overcome this limitation by dynamically adapting to the healing process [18]. These systems, which allow for gradual transfer of load to the bone as union progresses, reflect the growing recognition that fixation must evolve in harmony with the biological healing process.

2.4 Mechanobiology and flexible fixation

Recent biomechanical studies have demonstrated that flexible fixation, designed to meet physiological tension thresholds, stimulates osteogenic gene expression by increasing mechanotransduction [20, 21]. Hoang [4] demonstrated that mechanical tension regulates not only callus formation but also the differentiation of MSCs into osteoblasts via mechanosensitive signaling pathways such as YAP/TAZ and Wnt/β-catenin.

2.5 Fixation strategy and timing: The SDS model

When determining the fixation strategy for complex fractures, not only the fracture type but also the local soft-tissue condition and systemic host factors must be considered. In polytraumatized patients, systemic inflammation, metabolic disorders, or coagulopathy – frequently encountered in the early phase – may increase the risk of definitive fixation.

In this context, the SDS model, described by Kalbas et al. [3], offers a balanced approach bridging the gap between Early Total Care and Damage Control Orthopedics. The SDS model advocates that surgical timing should be based not on rigid time intervals but on the patient's physiological readiness.

In the presence of metabolic instability indicators, such as elevated lactate, acidosis, or hypothermia, temporary external fixation is preferred to allow systemic recovery; thereafter, definitive fixation is performed once stability and metabolic equilibrium are achieved. This patient-centered strategy has been shown to reduce mortality rates and significantly shorten intensive care unit stays compared with rigid early fixation protocols.

2.6 Imaging, 3D planning, and patient-specific implants

Once systemic stabilization is achieved, surgical planning becomes a process that demands precision and meticulous attention. Computed tomography with 3D reconstruction enables a detailed assessment of fracture morphology, guiding both preoperative decision-making and implant selection [5].

Liang et al. [5] reported that 3D printing technology allows the production of patient-specific anatomical plates and surgical guides, thereby increasing accuracy in reduction and screw placement while minimizing the need for intraoperative adjustments.

Ling et al. [6] demonstrated that 3D-assisted fracture surgery reduces intraoperative blood loss by approximately 30%, improves reduction accuracy by 20%, and shortens operative time. These patient-specific implants not only conform to the patient's anatomy but also preserve soft-tissue integrity, thereby reducing complication rates.

Collectively, these advances illustrate how digital engineering and additive manufacturing technologies are transforming trauma surgery from an intuition-driven art into a science grounded in precision and personalization.

2.7 Open fracture management: Early systemic intervention

The management of open fractures is a cornerstone of complex trauma care. These cases are complex injuries characterized by the simultaneous presence of mechanical destruction, soft tissue loss, and bacterial contamination. Infection prevention begins at the time of injury, not in the operating room. Whiting et al. [11] demonstrated that intravenous antibiotic administration within the first 60 minutes after trauma significantly reduces infection rates in open fractures. This finding clearly demonstrates the vital importance of early systemic intervention.

2.8 Debridement and "biological reconstruction"

However, antibiotic treatment alone is not sufficient. The most critical step in infection control is timely and complete surgical debridement. The goal of debridement is not only to remove contaminated tissue but also to biologically revitalize the wound. Metsemakers et al. [1] emphasized that debridement should be considered a form of "biological reconstruction" and that every surgical intervention should aim to transform the wound into a vascularized, living tissue environment. In this context, decisions such as which tissue to preserve, which to remove, and how to achieve tension-free closure directly impact infection control and ultimate healing [1].

2.9 Soft tissue reconstruction and timing

Soft tissue reconstruction is one of the most decisive stages of complex fracture treatment. Inadequate tissue coverage and persistent dead spaces are among the most significant causes of chronic infection. The modern orthoplastic approach, emphasized by Roberts et al. [13], integrates the disciplines of orthopedic and reconstructive surgery into a single, coordinated structure. It is recommended that definitive skeletal fixation and soft tissue closure should ideally be performed within the first 48 hours after injury; this principle is supported by both experimental and clinical data.

Negative pressure wound therapy (NPWT), while useful as a temporary bridging method, should not cause a delay in reconstruction. Local or free flap applications protect implants by restoring vascularity and creating a suitable biological environment for healing. This holistic approach has replaced the "fixation first, then closure" approach, which was historically associated with high infection rates.

2.10 FRI: Epidemiology, standards, and treatment algorithms

Despite all preventive measures, FRIs continue to occur in 2%–5% of long-bone injuries and up to 15% of open or revision cases. Rupp et al. [1] emphasized that achieving successful outcomes requires the use of standardized diagnostic criteria and unavoidable multidisciplinary collaboration.

The foundation of treatment consists of radical debridement, mechanical stabilization, and culture-directed antibiotic therapy. Li et al. [22] proposed a staged treatment algorithm that includes radical excision of infected tissue, temporary fixation when necessary, targeted systemic and local antibiotic administration, and delayed reconstruction after infection control has been achieved.

Metsemakers et al. [1] further argued that infection control should not be viewed as a separate phase of treatment but rather as an integral part of reconstruction. Their concept of "debridement equals reconstruction" underscores the importance of reestablishing biological continuity through healthy, well-vascularized tissue.

Complementing these contemporary treatment principles, Liu et al. [23] delineated several key risk factors that markedly increase susceptibility to deep surgical site infection in orthopedic trauma patients, including high-energy open fractures, prolonged operative duration, diabetes, obesity, and substantial soft-tissue compromise, thereby reinforcing the necessity of early risk stratification and rigorous preservation of the biological milieu during fixation.

2.11 Mechanical stability and antimicrobial strategies

Mechanical stability plays as critical a role as biological factors in the eradication of infection. Unstable fractures increase micromobility, fluid accumulation, and bacterial persistence, while stable fixation facilitates vascularization and immune cell access to the infected area [14]. Therefore, achieving both biological and mechanical stability is a decisive factor in infection control. Current applications include antibiotic-coated implants, reaming–irrigation–aspiration (RIA) systems, and dual plating techniques, aiming to simultaneously provide both mechanical stability and local antimicrobial defense [24]. This integrated approach demonstrates the level of biomechanical and microbiological knowledge achieved in trauma surgery.

2.12 Nonunion: Risk factors and individualized treatment

Despite substantial technological progress, nonunion and delayed union remain significant clinical challenges. Ghanem et al. [25] identified the primary risk factors associated with nonunion, including infection, metabolic disorders, malalignment, and smoking. Consequently, treatment strategies should be individualized according to the biological activity at the fracture site: enhancing stability in hypertrophic nonunions and stimulating biological activity in atrophic cases.

Autografts obtained through the RIA system provide abundant osteogenic material while minimizing donor-site morbidity. When autograft availability is limited, allografts or bone substitutes can serve as osteoconductive scaffolds. As noted by Bin Shahri et al. [16], the use of biological agents such as BMPs, PRP, and MSCs has markedly enhanced the surgeon's ability to modulate the biological environment. These agents promote angiogenesis, cellular differentiation, and osteogenesis, offering meaningful therapeutic benefits, particularly in resistant cases of nonunion [17].

Hoang et al. [4] further demonstrated that MSCs function not only as osteogenic precursor cells but also as potent immunomodulators. By regulating macrophage polarization and reducing chronic inflammation, MSCs create a regenerative microenvironment conducive to bone healing and consolidation [4].

2.13 Geriatric and osteoporotic fractures: Orthogeriatric management

Complex fractures in elderly and osteoporotic patients present an additional layer of therapeutic difficulty. Welzel et al. [17] reported an increasing incidence of fragility fractures in the aging population, characterized by poor bone quality and a high comorbidity burden. In this patient group, mechanical fixation alone is insufficient; simultaneous biological and systemic optimization is essential [17, 26, 27].

Pharmacologic agents, such as teriparatide and vitamin D supplementation, accelerate bone turnover and improve implant anchorage. Orthogeriatric care models involving geriatricians, physiotherapists, and nutritionists have been shown to reduce mortality and enhance postoperative mobility [28]. Welzel et al. [17] demonstrated that coordinated multidisciplinary management shortens hospital stays and improves independence scores at discharge.

Hutchinson et al. [14] further emphasized that frailty assessment and early mobilization programs play a decisive role in improving outcomes among geriatric trauma patients. Therefore, management in this population requires a holistic approach that integrates surgical intervention, rehabilitation, and metabolic optimization to restore function and preserve autonomy.

2.14 Technology–biology balance and surgical judgment

The evolution of complex fracture treatment represents a continuous transformation born from the intersection of innovative technologies and surgical experience. Computer-aided navigation, artificial intelligence (AI)-based fracture mapping, and 3D bioprinting technologies offer unprecedented levels of precision and customization in trauma surgery [6, 10]. However, lasting success still depends on understanding the fundamental biology of bone healing and respecting the host's physiological limits. Each fracture is unique, not only morphologically but also in its biological and systemic characteristics. Therefore, the modern orthopedic surgeon must adopt an approach that combines advanced technology with clinical intuition and surgical judgment, aiming to restore both anatomical integrity and functional capacity by balancing biology and mechanics [29].

3. Conclusion

3.1 Paradigm shift and holistic care

The evolution of complex fracture management has become a field shaped by the intersection of biology, biomechanics, and clinical reasoning. Once viewed as a mechanical problem reduced to the question of "how to fix broken bone fragments with the strongest possible structure," this process has now evolved into a multilayered discipline based on the principles of cellular physiology, vascular biology, infection control, and patient-specific optimization [14]. The modern trauma surgeon strives for functional restoration, prioritizing biological compatibility beyond rigid anatomical perfection. Through the integration of surgical precision, systemic optimization, and multidisciplinary collaboration, complex fracture management has evolved into a holistic care process extending from the moment of injury to the end of rehabilitation.

3.2 Infection control: Biological priorities

Recent research has clearly demonstrated that fracture healing is a biological process driven by the mechanical context. Rupp et al. [2] reported that even with the most advanced fixation systems, failure is inevitable when infection control and tissue protection are neglected. The foundation of successful reconstruction is preserving periosteal circulation, minimizing soft tissue trauma, and ensuring early vascular restoration. This principle is critical, especially in open and high-energy fractures, under the threat of bacterial contamination and ischemia.

Whiting et al. [11] and Roberts et al. [13] have shown that early antibiotic administration, timely debridement, and coordinated orthoplastic closure significantly reduce infection rates and the need for reoperation. Metsemakers et al. [1] emphasized the importance of standardized diagnostic criteria and a multidisciplinary approach for the management of FRI. These data suggest that infection prevention relies on the preservation of biological integrity, not technology.

3.3 Nonunion and delayed union: Orthobiologic support

Nonunion and delayed union remain among the principal challenges in the management of complex fractures. Ghanem et al. [25] and Impieri et al. [15] emphasized that biological failure frequently results from systemic disorders such as diabetes, smoking, malnutrition, and vitamin D deficiency. Therefore, the modern therapeutic approach must adopt a holistic model that encompasses not only mechanical fixation but also physiological optimization of the host.

While autografts and bone substitutes remain fundamental components of reconstruction, the introduction of orthobiologic agents such as BMPs, PRP, and MSCs has markedly accelerated biological healing. Bin Shahri et al. [16] reported that MSCs enhance bone regeneration by secreting osteogenic cytokines and promoting angiogenesis within the fracture gap.

Hoang et al. [4] further demonstrated that MSCs not only suppress inflammation but also modulate macrophage polarization toward the M2 phenotype, thereby creating a regenerative microenvironment that facilitates osteogenesis. These biologic agents accelerate callus formation, increase union rates, and shorten consolidation time, particularly in atrophic or infected nonunions [4].

3.4 Fixation philosophy and variable stiffness

Biological sensitivity has been a key determinant in the evolution of fixation philosophy. MIPO and bridging plating techniques offer better clinical outcomes by emphasizing indirect reduction and preserved soft tissue vascularity over extensive periosteal stripping and direct reduction. Locking plate systems, which function as internal fixators, provide angular stability while preserving periosteal circulation [18]. However, Bowers et al. [8] reported that excessively rigid fixation can slow healing by inhibiting the micromobility necessary for callus maturation. Therefore, variable stiffness implant systems aim to dynamically adapt to the healing process and gradually transfer load to the bone.

3.5 Timing and physiological preparation (SDS)

This approach is consistent with the biological reality that bone remodeling requires controlled tension. The SDS concept, developed by Kalbas et al. [3], demonstrates that surgical timing should be determined not by a fixed time but rather by the patient's physiological preparation level. This patient-centered approach has improved outcomes in polytrauma patients by reducing complications, inflammatory responses, and the length of intensive care stay.

3.6 Digital technologies and a personalized approach

Digital technologies also support this biological and personalized approach. Liang et al. [5] demonstrated that the production of patient-specific plates and surgical guides using 3D printing technology improves anatomical fit and shortens surgical time. Ling et al. [6] reported a 30% improvement in blood loss and a 20% improvement in reduction accuracy with 3D-assisted surgery. Castillón et al. [7] demonstrated that establishing biomechanical continuity between new and old implants in previously implanted bones reduces stress concentration and lowers the risk of re-fracture.

3.7 Multidisciplinary collaboration and its impact on outcomes

A multidisciplinary approach has become an essential component of modern trauma care. Hutchinson et al. [14] demonstrated that structured team meetings involving orthopedics, plastic surgery, infectious diseases, and geriatrics specialists in shared decision-making processes improve both early surgical decisions and long-term functional outcomes. Similarly, Rupp et al. [2] reported that regular multidisciplinary assessments reduce the rates of recurrent infections and reoperations.

In conclusion, the current state of complex fracture management is a holistic synthesis of biological sensitivity, mechanical accuracy, and interdisciplinary collaboration. The fundamental principles of twenty-first-century orthopedics are based on "respecting biology, rebuilding mechanics, and integrating care." The modern orthopedic surgeon should view every fracture not merely as a mechanical failure but as a biological event within a living organism, utilizing technology as a tool to enhance the balance and harmony of biology and clinical judgment.

Acknowledgments

The author thanks the Orthopedics and Traumatology Department of Elmalı State Hospital for their academic and clinical support during the preparation of this chapter.

Special appreciation is extended to colleagues who contributed through critical discussions and case sharing, which helped refine the concepts presented herein.

No external funding was received for this work.

Conflict of Interest

The author declares no conflict of interest.

DOI: http://dx.doi.org/10.5772/intechopen.1014248

Abbreviations

3D	Three-dimensional
AI	Artificial intelligence
BMP	Bone morphogenetic protein
FRI	Fracture-related infection
MIPO	Minimally invasive percutaneous plate osteosynthesis
MSCs	Mesenchymal stem cells
NPWT	Negative pressure wound therapy
PRP	Platelet-rich plasma
RIA	Reaming–irrigation–aspiration
SDS	Safe definitive surgery
TGF-β	Transforming growth factor beta
VEGF	Vascular endothelial growth factor
MDT	Multidisciplinary team

Appendices and Nomenclature

No appendices are included in this chapter. Abbreviations used throughout the text are listed in the abbreviations section.

Author details

Murat Yüncü
Department of Orthopaedics and Traumatology, Elmalı State Hospital, Antalya, Türkiye

*Address all correspondence to: muratyuncu1@gmail.com

References

[1] Metsemakers WJ, Morgenstern M, Senneville E, Borens O, Govaert GAM, Onsea J, et al. General treatment principles for fracture-related infection: Recommendations from an international expert group. Archives of Orthopaedic and Trauma Surgery. 2020;**140**:1013–1027

[2] Rupp M, Walter N, Popp D, Hitzenbichler F, Heyd R, Geis S, et al. Multidisciplinary treatment of fracture-related infection has a positive impact on clinical outcome—A retrospective case control study at a tertiary referral center. Antibiotics. 2023;**12**:230

[3] Kalbas Y, Heining SM, Kaiser A, Klingebiel FKL, Pfeifer R, Wanner GA, et al. Fracture fixation in polytraumatized patients-From an interdisciplinary early total/appropriate care to the safe definitive surgery concept. Frontiers in Medicine (Lausanne). 2024:11. DOI: 10.3389/FMED.2024.1362986

[4] Hoang DM, Pham PT, Bach TQ, Ngo ATL, Nguyen QT, Phan TTK, et al. Stem cell-based therapy for human diseases. Signal Transduction and Targeted Therapy. 2022:7. DOI: 10.1038/S41392-022-01134-4

[5] Liang H, Chen B, Duan S, Yang L, Xu R, Zhang H, et al. Treatment of complex limb fractures with 3D printing technology combined with personalized plates: A retrospective study of case series and literature review. Frontiers in Surgery. 2024:11. DOI: 10.3389/FSURG.2024.1383401/FULL

[6] Ling K, Wang W, Liu J. Current developments in 3D printing technology for orthopedic trauma: A review. Medicine. 2025;**104**:e41946. DOI: 10.1097/MD.0000000000041946

[7] Castillón P, Vives JMM, Aguado HJ, Agundez AC, Ortega-Briones A, Núñez JH. Consensus review on peri-implant femur fracture treatment: Peri-Implant Spanish Consensus (PISCO) investigators' recommendations. EFORT Open Reviews. 2024;**9**:40–50. DOI: 10.1530/EOR-23-0105

[8] Bowers KM, Anderson DE. Delayed union and nonunion: Current concepts, prevention, and correction: A review. Bioengineering (Basel). 2024;11. DOI: 10.3390/BIOENGINEERING11060525

[9] Wang C, Li C. Early weight-bearing after ankle fracture surgery: A systematic review and meta-analysis of functional outcomes and safety. Journal of Orthopaedic Surgery and Research. 2025;**20**. DOI: 10.1186/S13018-025-06216-X

[10] Mohamed A, Elasad A, Fuad U, Pengas I, Elsayed A, Bhamidipati P, et al. Artificial intelligence in trauma and orthopaedic surgery: A comprehensive review from diagnosis to rehabilitation. Cureus. 2025;**17**. DOI: 10.7759/CUREUS.92280

[11] Whiting PS, Obremskey W, Johal H, Shearer D, Volgas D, Balogh ZJ. Open fractures: Evidence-based best practices. OTA International. 2024;7. DOI: 10.1097/OI9.0000000000000313

[12] Li D, Li J, Xu Y, Ling C, Qiu Y, Zhu Z, et al. Topical vancomycin powder for the prevention of surgical site infections in spinal deformity surgery: A systematic review and meta-analysis. European Spine Journal.

2024;**33**(12):4653–4663. DOI: 10.1007/S00586-024-08494-1

[13] Roberts L, Radwan Ahmed M, Agrawal D K. Current strategies in the prevention and management of infection in open fractures. Journal of Orthopaedics and Sports Medicine. 2025;7:218–229. DOI: 10.26502/JOSM.511500198

[14] Hutchinson K, Bretherton CB, Gmati A, Handley B. Multidisciplinary management of orthopaedic trauma - are we adhering to the guidelines? The Annals of the Royal College of Surgeons of England. 2025;**107**: 217–222. DOI: 10.1308/RCSANN.2024.0048

[15] Impieri L, Pezzi A, Hadad H, Peretti GM, Mangiavini L, Rossi N. Orthobiologics in delayed union and non-union of adult long bones fractures: A systematic review. Bone Reports. 2024;21. DOI: 10.1016/j.bonr.2024.101760

[16] Bin Shahri N, Chong AKS, Karjalainen T. The role of orthobiologics in bone healing and joint and tendon degeneration in the upper limb. Journal of Hand Surgery (European Volume). 2025;50:728–737. DOI: 10.1177/17531934251327034

[17] Welzel L, Omar M, Müller CW. Complications following surgical treatment of ankle fractures in the elderly: Can they be avoided? Orthop Rev (Pavia). 2024;16. DOI: 10.52965/001C.116370

[18] Barwar N, Gargi G, Rai A, Elhence A, Banerjee S, Gahlot N. Dual plating in the management of nonunion complex distal femur fractures following lateral locked plate fixation: Radiological and functional outcomes of a prospective study. Journal of Trauma and Injury. 2025;**38**:125–136. DOI: 10.20408/JTI.2024.0054

[19] Beeharry MW, Ahmad B. Principles of fracture healing and fixation: A literature review. Cureus. 2024;**16**. DOI: 10.7759/CUREUS.76250

[20] Gardner MJ, van der Meulen MCH, Demetrakopoulos D, Wright TM, Myers ER, Bostrom MP. In vivo cyclic axial compression affects bone healing in the mouse tibia. Journal of Orthopaedic Research. 2006;**24**: 1679–1686. DOI: 10.1002/JOR.20230

[21] Ma Q, Miri Z, Haugen HJ, Moghanian A, Loca D. Significance of mechanical loading in bone fracture healing, bone regeneration, and vascularization. Journal of Tissue Engineering. 2023;14. DOI: 10.1177/20417314231172573

[22] Li C, Foster AL, Han NHB, Trampuz A, Schuetz M. A bibliometric analysis of clinical research on fracture-related infection. BioMed Research International. 2022;**2022**. DOI: 10.1155/2022/8171831

[23] Liu H, Wang Y, Xing H, Chang Z, Pan J. Risk factors for deep surgical site infections following orthopedic trauma surgery: A meta-analysis and systematic review. Journal of Orthopaedic Surgery and Research. 2024;**19**. DOI: 10.1186/S13018-024-05299-2

[24] Landrino M, Alberio RL, Clemente A, Grassi FA. The Reamer-Irrigator-Aspirator (RIA) system for the treatment of aseptic femoral nonunions: Report of two cases and literature review. Orthop Rev (Pavia). 2022;**14**:37889. DOI: 10.52965/001c.37889

[25] Ghanem W, Ezzeddine H, Saad R, Kiwan E, Dahdouh R, Fakih O, et al. State of the Nonunion: A review of the latest literature. Orthop Rev (Pavia). 2025:17. DOI: 10.52965/001C.129085

[26] Orji C, Ojo C, Onobun DE, Igbokwe K, Khaliq F, Ononye R. Fracture non-union in osteoporotic bones: Current practice and future directions. Cureus. 2024;**16**. DOI: 10.7759/CUREUS.69778

[27] Pankratz C, Risch A, Oxen J, Cintean R, Boehringer A, Gebhard F, et al. Orthogeriatric care-outcome of different fragility fractures. Archives of Orthopaedic and Trauma Surgery. 2023;**143**:6641–6647

[28] Van Heghe A, Mordant G, Dupont J, Dejaeger M, Laurent MR, Gielen E. Effects of orthogeriatric care models on outcomes of hip fracture patients: A systematic review and meta-analysis. Calcified Tissue International. 2022;**110**:162–184. DOI: 10.1007/S00223-021-00913-5/TABLES/6

[29] Rupp M, Walter N, Bärtl S, Heyd R, Hitzenbichler F, Alt V. Fracture-related infection-epidemiology, etiology, diagnosis, prevention, and treatment. Deutsches Arzteblatt International. 2024;**121**:17–24. DOI: 10.3238/ARZTEBL.M2023.0233